Dr. Miriam Stoppard's
BOOK OF
BABY CARE

Dr. Miriam Stoppard's
BOOK OF
BABY CARE

New York   1977   **Atheneum**

Library of Congress Cataloging in Publication Data
Stoppard, Miriam.
  Dr. Miriam Stoppard's Book of baby care.

  Includes index.
    1. Infants — Care and hygiene. 2. Pregnancy.
I. Title. II. Title: Book of baby care.
RJ61.S8946   649'.122   77–76668
ISBN 0–689–10810–9

Composition by Dix Typesetting Co.,
    Syracuse, New York
Printed and bound by The Murray Printing Company,
    Forge Village, Massachusetts
First American Edition

For Oliver, Barnaby, William, and Edmund

Preface

The baby-care world is not short of experts. Much of the information in this book is the received wisdom of years of pediatric study and practice, and beyond the field of medicine itself there are yet more experts with theories on everything from breakfast foods to thumb-sucking. But when I was in clinical practice and saw a baby with a problem, whether physiological or behavioral, I learned never to underestimate the opinion of the caring parent.

Before your baby is a month old you will know things about that baby that no book can tell you. If I came and sat on your bookshelf in person, I could not tell you some of the things you could tell me — whether the note in his cry, for instance, means his bottle nipple is blocked, or that he is getting sick, or just that he needs changing. Expertise is about textbook babies, parenthood is about *your* baby.

So let me tell you what this book is not. It is not a book of rules, and still less is it the baby equivalent of a service manual. It is not a set of solutions to a set of problems, nor is it a set of instructions.

It is, however, an attempt to guide you in making *your* rules. To give you the latest information on aspects of baby care that are matters of medical fact. To give you the benefit of one doctor/ mother's experience that will apply to all babies some of the time, and to some babies all of the time. In short, to give you a background against which you can liberate your parental instincts and your common sense.

Lastly, almost every baby will at some time need the kind of medical help that you can't get from a book. My hope for this book is that it will give you the confidence to know immediately when that help is needed — and the confidence to know and enjoy the times when all the family are doing fine.

Acknowledgments

Author's Acknowledgments

I should like to thank Dr. Elizabeth Bryan, a friend and pediatrician who commented on each chapter as I wrote it; Dr. David Harvey of Queen Charlotte's Hospital, London, who was the first person to read the book in its entirety and who made very helpful suggestions; my secretary, Mrs. Margaret Hornby, who gave up her free time to type the text; my husband, Tom, who encouraged me to start writing the book in the first place; and all my children for their unwitting contributions.

Picture Acknowledgments

Photographs and illustrations are supplied by or reproduced by kind permission of the following:

Andra Nelki 45 (left and right), 61, 101 (bottom left and top right)
Barnaby's Picture Library 95 (bottom right), 98 (bottom left), 99 (top), 103 (bottom right)
Department of Medical Illustration, Birmingham Children's Hospital 102 (bottom left)
Prof. R. Illingworth, Sheffield Children's Hospital 92, 93 (bottom), 94 (top), 95 (top left), 96 (top)
Marshall Cavendish 99 (bottom), 93 (bottom)
Martin Haydon 103 (bottom right)
National Childbirth Trust 52, 53
The Observer, courtesy of Transworld Features Syndicate 19
Private Collection 96 (bottom left)
Rex Features 40
The remaining pictures were supplied by Raymond Irons.

Contents

Dr. Miriam Stoppard's

BOOK OF
BABY CARE

1 Conception

It may seem odd to begin a book on baby care with *conceiving* the baby. But there are good reasons for doing so. Though we start counting a baby's age from the day it is born, strictly speaking a baby has been growing and developing for the previous nine months in an environment that is entirely created by its mother. Probably at no other time in life are we so completely controlled by another being, by what it is doing, by what it is feeling (oh, yes, if the mother is happy the baby almost certainly feels it), even by what it is eating. A whole set of habits, a whole metabolism is impressed upon us. By the time a baby is born you might say it has had the initial programing which will affect its physical and psychological future. Not only that, but at an even earlier stage (fertilization) it was formed from a single cell that contained a component from each of its parents: it was 'fingerprinted' in their image. For this reason pediatricians are currently suggesting that the care of children should start not with the birth of the baby but with the union of its parents. Or even further back, when the future pediatric patient is minus five years old. How far back can we go now? To conception.

If asked, I am sure most of us would say that one way or another we can largely control the act of conceiving for ourselves. This may not be so. Most lower animals have a breeding season; we would rather believe we have not. Man is the only animal that eats when he is not hungry, drinks when he is not thirsty, and makes love at all seasons. It comes as something of a shock, therefore, to find that in many countries the season has a great deal to do with conception in human beings; and that conception itself may be controlled by the same physiological mechanisms as in animals.

In the United States the peak months for conception are October and November. This would seem a reasonable natural precaution, as children born in July and August will have the benefit of warm weather during their first weeks of life. In England and Wales, Sweden and West Germany, it's the other way about, with a peak in

3

the summer months. Further research has shown that, in the northern hemisphere at least, the conception rate varies roughly with the temperature. And the peaks swing from winter to summer as you move from the warmer to the colder countries. The conception peak normally occurs when the monthly average temperature is about 20°C (68°F). In nearly all countries the annual low point is around March, and this prompted the statisticians to look for influences such as social conventions. A glance at a calendar reminded them that March is the time of Lent and Easter, during which time religious considerations, particularly among Roman Catholics, impose a degree of self-denial.

Animals can be made to extend their breeding season by several weeks if they are exposed to six hours of extra light a day. Can we be similarly affected by changes in our environment? Well, some very clever research carried out in southern England suggests we may be. A group of general practitioners who examined the number of births month by month in relation to the daily hours of sunshine found that, irrespective of the time of year, conception is more likely to occur on those days when there is more than average sunshine.

Leaving aside speculation, there are less intriguing but infinitely more basic biological factors directing the timing of conception. On a quite different time scale, the most important factor is that a woman is fertile or capable of conceiving for only a few days of any twenty-eight or so. These are the days around ovulation, which is generally in the middle of the monthly cycle. But for a woman who does not menstruate strictly every four weeks, it is more accurately fourteen to sixteen days before her period starts, regardless of the length of her cycle. It is possible for her to detect the day of ovulation by taking her temperature every day, for on ovulation day it rises and stays up for the rest of the month. If she repeats this for several months a fairly constant pattern emerges. It's not absolutely foolproof — some women have been known to conceive while menstruating — but it is a good guide. The information can be used two ways; it not only tells her when to have intercourse but when *not* to have it, as the high-temperature days constitute the 'unsafe period.'

Is it possible to have a baby of the sex you want? In the past, boys were always more highly prized than girls, and ancient writings are full of helpful suggestions on how to have a boy. As long ago as 500 BC it was suggested that a woman should lie on her right side while making love in order to have a boy. Some communities believe in holding the right testicle or nibbling the right ear during intercourse. Biologically, however, only the father is responsible for the baby's sex. Men produce sperm of two types — Y sperm, which produce boys, and X sperm, which produce girls. The ovum, the woman's contribution to a new child, is biologically sexless. If we can find out something about the behavior of X and Y sperm we might be able to use the knowledge in the hope of getting a baby of the sex we want. We already know quite a lot: male sperm are smaller, faster, stronger and shorter lived than the female sperm. They prefer a less acid environment than female sperm. The acid conditions in the vagina therefore marginally favor female sperm. Based on these facts, but on very little scientific confirmation by actual results, some doctors make the following suggestions for producing male children:

   1. Have intercourse on or as near to ovulation as possible. (The faster male sperm will reach the egg before the heavy, slow, female sperm.)
   2. Have a period of abstinence before. (This increases the proportion of male sperm present.)
   3. Douche with a solution of bicarbonate of soda — one teaspoon to one pint of water (to make the vagina more favorable to male sperm) prior to intercourse.

Conversely, this may work for a girl:

   1. Stop intercourse two or three days before ovulation. (Male sperm will die, leaving only female sperm for fertilization.)
   2. Do not abstain. (This lowers the proportion of male sperm.)
   3. Douche with weak vinegar solution — one part vinegar to ten parts water (acid favors female sperm) before intercourse.

Fertilization

Fertilization occurs when the ovary liberates a ripe ovum which is subsequently penetrated by a sperm. The egg and the sperm have gone through a lot before this mating. The ovum has been waiting along with a half a million or so others since the mother's birth for its turn to mature and burst out of the surface of the ovary, to drop into and traverse the abdominal cavity and to find its way into the Fallopian tube. Once safely there it is wafted along the tube by small hairs toward the uterus.

If sperm are present, the ovum is fertilized about a third of the way along the tube. This sperm has had quite a journey; it has been traveling for two weeks inside the man's body from the depths of the testis; only seconds before ejaculation it becomes mobile, so that the lashings of its whip-like tail can carry it at top speed beyond the hostile, acid conditions of the vagina to the cervix; here it climbs the 'silken ladder' formed by the secretions in the neck of the uterus; without pause it treks through the cavernous body of the uterus until it reaches the ovum. Once in the vicinity of the relatively huge ovum, sperm are chemically drawn to it and attach themselves like limpets over the whole surface. Finally one sperm, usually a latecomer, pierces the outer coat of the ovum. Instantaneously the egg loses its attraction and all the superfluous spermatozoa fall back.

Ejaculation to fertilization may take only one hour. In that time the sperm has covered a distance thousands of times its own length. It is crucial that sperm are capable of making this sprint. The ripe ovum can probably only survive for twelve hours, maximum twenty-four, and sperm retain the power to fertilize for not longer than twenty-four hours after being released into the vagina. Conception is therefore unlikely unless coitus occurs one or two days before, or immediately after, ovulation.

Only the head of the sperm actually fuses with the ovum to form a single cell — the superfluous body and tail are lost. This cell,

OPPOSITE: The female reproductive system from the front. The sperms travel up through the uterus and along the Fallopian tube to meet the ovum which has been released from the ovary during ovulation. Enlarged detail (1) shows the ovum immediately prior to ovulation. (2) shows fertilization — one sperm has penetrated the ovum. As the fertilized ovum travels along the Fallopian tube toward the uterus it undergoes mitotic division to form two, then four, then eight cells and so on (3) (4), which results in the formation of a ball of cells (5) and these will develop into the future embryo (6). The growing embryo becomes implanted (7) in the uterus wall about twelve days after fertilization. Here it can obtain food and continue to develop.

FEMALE REPRODUCTIVE SYSTEM FROM THE SIDE

ovary
uterus
pubic bone
clitoris
labium
vagina
bladder
cervix
rectum and anus

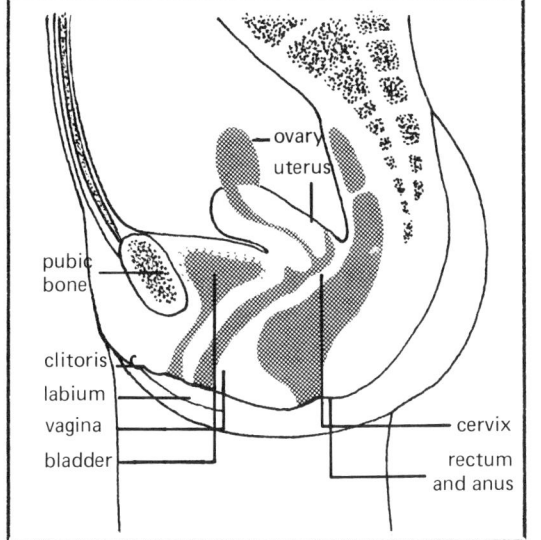

MALE REPRODUCTIVE SYSTEM FROM THE SIDE

bladder
pubic bone
prostate
seminal vesicle
epididymis
testis
erectile spongy tissue
rectum and anus

FEMALE REPRODUCTIVE SYSTEM FROM THE FRONT

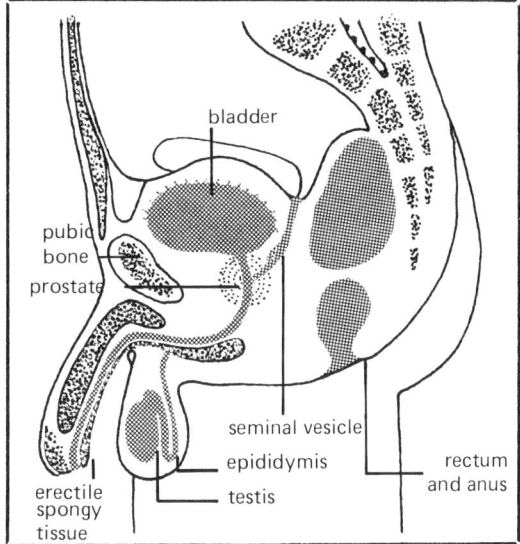

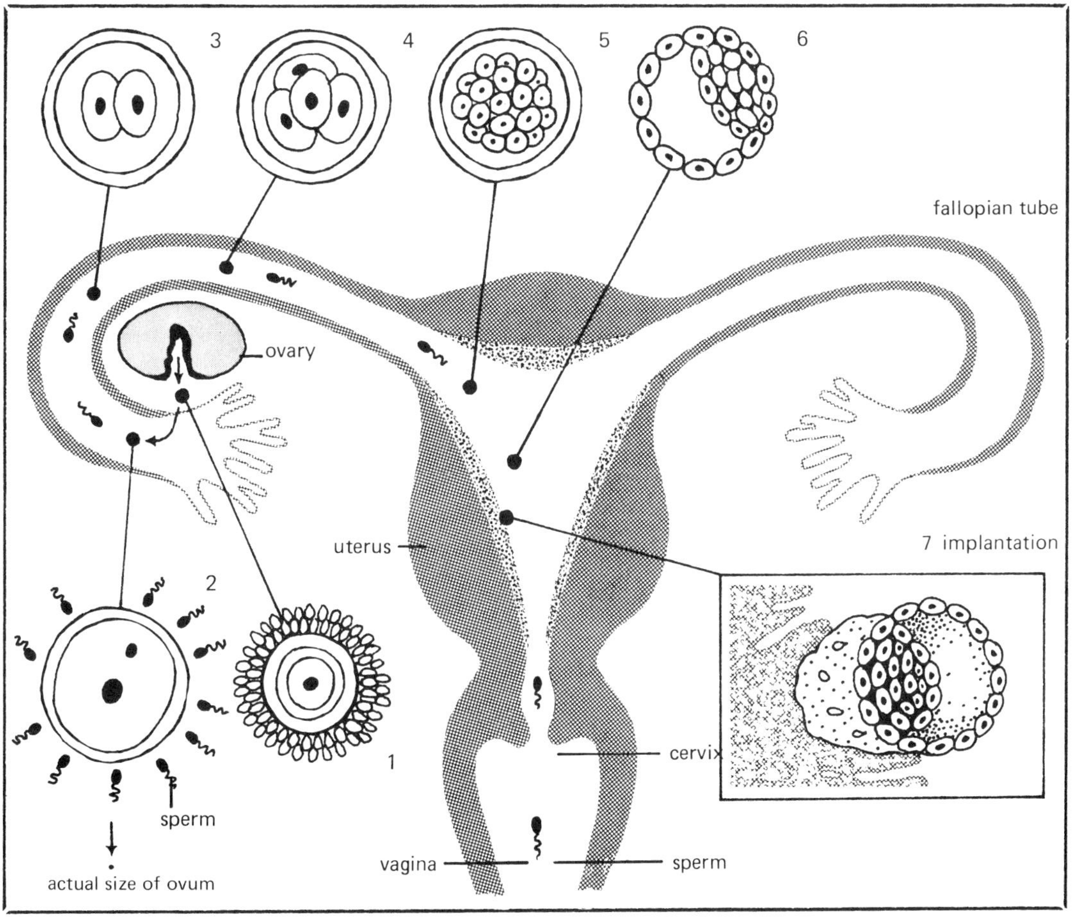

3
4
5
6
fallopian tube
ovary
uterus
7 implantation
2
1
cervix
sperm
actual size of ovum
vagina
sperm

with a contribution from each parent, gets down to the business of producing a new organism immediately, and divides into two in the first twenty-four hours. By the fourth day it is a round ball of cells and has reached the uterus, where it floats free for another two or three days in a nutritious 'milk' secreted by glands in the womb. About the seventh day it attaches itself to the wall of the uterus and then burrows deep into the lining, until by the twenty-first or twenty-second day of the menstrual cycle the developing embryo is firmly embedded (or implanted), with its point of entry safely sealed off. Just about the time a period is due, the tiny fetus has formed a physical union with the mother. It is continuously bathed in a lake of her blood and this facilitates the passage of food and waste to and from the embryo.

The most fruitful parasitic relationship in biology has begun.

Miscarriage

For many women this union between mother and embryo resists any attempt at disruption, but miscarriages do occur and it is difficult to get accurate figures about their frequency. Some, if they happen early, go undetected; many, if detected, are unreported. In the first few weeks, even if detected, they are difficult to confirm and it may be that early miscarriages occur very frequently. It is said that up to a third of all first pregnancies miscarry, but nevertheless a normal second pregnancy usually ensues. The theory is that the womb needs a trial run in order to become fully developed. Excluding early unrecognized miscarriages and those that are procured, miscarriage occurs in something like one in ten of all pregnancies. As women get older this figure probably rises to as high as one in five. The vast majority of diagnosable miscarriages occur before the twelfth week of pregnancy — in fact 80 percent occur during the second and third months.

There are so many possible causes of miscarriage (and several may operate at one time) that without special investigation it is usually not possible to find a definite cause. This upsets many women who, suffering from feelings of inadequacy and failure, cast around for something to blame. It is some comfort if a miscarriage can be seen as a necessary safeguard against having abnormal babies, for by far the most frequent single cause is an abnormality of the developing embryo. Between half to three-quarters of early miscarriages occur for this reason. The commonest causes of malformation are chromosomal abnormalities, then virus infections of the mother, for instance German measles, and certain drugs. It is a good rule not to take even over-the-counter medicines once pregnancy is suspected.

If the mother is healthy and strong there is very little that will disturb a pregnancy. Most pregnant women, contrary to folklore, are impervious to frights, emotional upsets, accidents, purgatives, quinine, and even operations. Indeed curettage (scraping the womb) has been carried out inadvertently when the patient was pregnant, and the pregnancy has continued normally. There are undoubtedly, however, a very few women who are miscarriage prone, and any of the factors mentioned above may precipitate miscarriage in these women.

The old-fashioned method of treatment for a threatened miscarriage (that is, if bleeding occurs) meant confinement to bed; sedatives were given to calm the mother, and occasionally female hormones, in particular the pregnancy hormone progesterone. As none of the treatments has been proved valuable, and as a malformed embryo so often sets off miscarriage, the modern approach involves nothing more than taking things easy. It gives just as good results as any other treatment. Roughly three-quarters of women who threaten to miscarry, however, go on to produce a normal healthy child. Only about a quarter inevitably miscarry because they have a deformed embryo. At most, five in a hundred subsequently miscarry for other reasons.

There are a few women who habitually miscarry, but the statistics are encouraging. About two-thirds of all women who have miscarried as many as three times go on to a normal fourth pregnancy without any special treatment. Nonetheless, the more miscarriages a woman has, the less likely it is that they have occurred by chance. Three consecutive miscarriages are now generally accepted as requiring special investigation and treatment.

Low Fertility

When I was a medical student, the Professor of Obstetrics and Gynecology introduced his subject by saying, "Obstetrics are largely the problem of having too many children or too few." To begin with the latter problem: approximately one in twenty couples in the United States is subfertile and is unable to have babies. In many women the desire for children can be intense, overriding considerations of a slim figure or the pursuit of a career. Childlessness can be something of an emotional upset to a woman and may not only result in unhappiness and strained relations with her husband, but also in unaccountable headaches, fatigue, exhaustion, depression or insomnia.

The investigation of a couple's apparent infertility with its anatomical and hormonal booby traps is difficult enough, but first it must be discussed, usually with the family doctor. Essentially, couples must bring to these discussions the willingness to be guided and to be realistic. In a recent survey about 5 percent of couples seeking help at an infertility clinic expected a prescription for a fertility pill without any investigation, while others were unwilling to involve their partner in the investigation. The first step is the acceptance that low fertility is not a matter of either partner exclusively, but of the couple as a unit. For fertility is relative to each couple and few people are completely sterile or fully fertile. Seen in this way the fertility of a couple is the sum of the fertilities of the partners. The high fertility of one can to some degree compensate for the low fertility of the other. On the other hand, marginal fertility in both partners may result in sterility. This explains the paradox of a childless couple splitting up and *both* producing children without difficulty with a new partner.

About 15 percent of marriages in most western countries are childless. The figure for *sterile* marriages is somewhat lower, for the higher figure includes those couples beyond the reproductive age and those who deliberately avoid pregnancy. However there is useful information on this question from a survey done in England and Wales between 1900 and 1909, when only a few couples used any form of contraception; nearly twelve out of every hundred couples were childless at the end of ten years. An important factor turned out to be the woman's age at the time of her marriage — the older she was, the greater the chance that her marriage would be sterile. Nowadays about 8 percent of couples young enough to have children and wanting them go childless.

Fertility in women is certainly affected by age and begins to diminish around the age of twenty-five. The chances of conception for your age are indicated here:

Less than 20 years of age:	95 percent
20–25:	94 percent
26–30:	89 percent
31–35:	83 percent
35–40:	70 percent

The decline in a man's fertility is more gradual, being the same as a woman's at the age of twenty and waning slowly to 10 percent at the age of sixty.

There is an increased risk of mongolism in a baby produced by a mother over the age of forty. As a rule a woman of this age should talk things over with her doctor before embarking on a pregnancy, especially if it's her first pregnancy. For some reason we don't yet understand, there is an increased risk of an abnormal baby if the mother is less than sixteen years old at term — i.e. due to go into labor. The 'elderly primagravida' is a woman over the age of thirty-five having her first child, and she is likely to have a slightly longer labor than her younger friends. Roughly speaking, labor increases in length by about one to two hours for every ten years of age, though many women over the age of forty have easy labors even with their first baby. Never be put off from starting a pregnancy because of your age, but be meticulous about your prenatal care.

Having picked a way through the long list of causes, all of which may be eliminated, one of the most sensitive problems to deal with is left — the psychological and emotional barriers to fertility. Understandably many people find this subject difficult and embarrassing and it may be necessary to seek help from a marriage counselor or psychiatrist. Unless psychological and emotional disharmony is obvious, leading to avoidance of intercourse — dyspareunia (pain on intercourse), where feelings of distaste or fear cause tightening of the vaginal muscles; or difficulty in maintaining an erection or premature ejaculation — physical or hormonal causes are sought first. Close questioning of the couple may reveal past illnesses that could affect their fertility, like a previous genital injury, or infection with mumps, or x-ray exposure to the lower abdomen in the man, peritonitis or pelvic infection or an illegal abortion (which is complicated by infection or physical damage) in the woman, or venereal disease in either partner. All these may contribute to low fertility.

There are two main causes of infertility in men — a blockage in the tubes between the testis and the penis and inadequate production of sperm. Blockage is normally due to one of three things — injury, infection, or failure of the ducts to develop normally prior to birth. Inadequate sperm production involves three kinds of deficiency — a low sperm count (even though 'low' still means millions of sperm in a drop of semen), low sperm mobility, and large numbers of abnormal sperm. These characteristics must be examined in the man *and the woman* after intercourse.

Full-scale investigation of a woman's infertility involves complicated biochemical tests, special x-rays, even surgical exploration and keeping daily records of her menstrual cycle; so it is frequently a time-consuming and lengthy process and is usually undertaken only by specialists in the field. The failure to ovulate or produce sufficient numbers of sperm is amenable to stimulation by drugs; in fact the same chemicals can be used in both men and women, though results are much better in women. At first a fairly simple drug is used in gradually increasing dosage until ovulation occurs regularly. If this initial treatment fails, hormonal treatment is considered, though there are explicit guidelines for doctors to help them decide which patients will benefit. Pregnancy results in about two-thirds of patients who receive this form of therapy, and in a comparatively short time — about three to four months. With so much experience of careful dosage adjustment, multiple pregnancies are becoming rarer, and in a recent study only 5 percent produced twins or triplets. Miscarriages do occur in these induced pregnancies, at a rate of something like one in eight.

Couples should be aware that setting out on a chain of investigations and treatment which may be unsuccessful is likely to cause emotional tension and sexual frustration. This may strain a marriage more than childlessness. There is no point in treating infertility if the result is a fertile couple who cannot stand each other.

2 Pregnancy

Pregnancy is a unique state; unlike all other situations where nature tries to correct the slightest disturbance of the equilibrium, in pregnancy the seesaw is allowed to tip heavily in favor of the baby, and the mother's body makes any change or sacrifice necessary for its healthy growth. These changes occur mainly in the early part of pregnancy and are designed not only to anticipate any possible demands of the embryo when it is in the womb, but also to provide for it after birth by laying in stores of fat and minerals that can later be converted to milk for breast-feeding.

Traditionally pregnancy is said to last, on average, nine calendar months and one week, and can be split up into three periods of three months, known as trimesters. It is not just the time factor that makes it convenient to punctuate pregnancy in this way; it is also medically rational, as there are certain events which commonly occur in relation to only one of the trimesters. Pregnancy sickness, for instance, is largely confined to the first; high blood pressure is rarely a problem until the third.

The development of the baby can also be divided into three stages, but on quite a different time scale; the first stage is from fertilization to successful implantation — a matter of days; the second is from here to the end of the eighth week when all the vital organs have begun to take form; the eighth week to the end of pregnancy can be seen as the third stage — the growth spurt of the fully formed embryo.

Diagnosis and Dates

The commonest cause of amenorrhea, or failure to menstruate, is pregnancy, and the classic sign of pregnancy is amenorrhea. However, the diagnosis of pregnancy is not always straightforward and depends on information from several sources, so in the early weeks it is almost impossible to diagnose pregnancy by examination alone.

13

At six weeks there are certain changes that can be picked up by an observant doctor, such as a slight bluish tinge in the wall of the vagina, a slight softening of the cervix and a very slight enlargement of the uterus, but no physician would rely on these signs alone. Just as helpful are changes that the woman will have noticed in herself, such as her breasts becoming tender and tingling occasionally, feeling nauseated if not actually being sick, needing to empty the bladder more frequently than before and experiencing overwhelming fatigue — the inability to eat, even smile, from tiredness — and the tendency to drop into a deep sleep within seconds of sitting down. Somewhere between eight and twelve weeks the uterus does become large enough to feel, but nowadays there are simple, quick, but nonetheless reliable laboratory tests to confirm pregnancy, which require only a specimen of urine. They become positive twelve days after the first day of the missed period and can be performed in two minutes; a positive test is 99 percent certain.

Pregnancy generally lasts 266 days from conception. The expected delivery date can be more easily calculated, however, if the duration of pregnancy is taken as being 280 days (nine calendar months and one week) from the first day of the last period. An alternative calculation involves subtracting three months from the first day of the last period and then adding 7 days. For example, if the first day of the last is September 12, the expected date of delivery is June 12, add 7 days . . . June 19 of the next year. This represents an average of course, and depends on your being able to remember precisely when a period started (it really is worth putting it in your diary) and on having regular 28-day cycles. Many women do not have 28-day cycles and so babies are born quite normally any time between thirty-nine and forty-one weeks. Pregnancies which appear to be much shorter or longer than this probably represent miscalculated dates. For instance, some women experience a short bleed at period time after they have conceived. Were this considered the last period, pregnancy would appear four weeks shorter than its actual length.

Care of the Mother

REST

Obviously you should get as much rest as you can, but there are not many women in the happy position of being able to lie down every afternoon for two hours. It is not necessary to have compulsory rest periods — it is enough to adapt your normal pattern of activity and rest when you can. A naturally active woman will probably want to stay quite active and she should do what she wants as long as she does not become overtired. For once in your life take seriously the advice, 'Don't stand when you can sit, don't sit when you can lie.'

SLEEP

Oddly enough many pregnant women, though able to fall asleep easily, often wake a few hours later and cannot get back to sleep. A good night's sleep is important though, and you should consult your doctor if you have a problem getting sufficient rest.

EXERCISE

Whether you are at home or at business you will get enough exercise going about your normal day. Walking is good for you but you should stop and rest if you feel tired. Swimming will exercise all the muscles of the body, particularly the abdomen, and if you are a strong swimmer there is little danger in swimming in a warm pool as late as the seventh month. Cycling is the same. But from the very early months on it is foolhardy to ride horseback, downhill ski or water-ski — for one thing you cannot balance properly or move fast, and for another it is impossible to anticipate accidents. If any lifting has to be done you should squat where possible and avoid bending.

TRAVEL

There is no danger specific to pregnancy in any form of travel — no, not even flying, though most doctors would prefer you not to take the risk after the seventh month. Recent research suggests that you should avoid going up mountains above a height of ten thousand feet during early pregnancy, as the fetus may suffer damage. It would be taking an unnecessary risk, however, to travel far from home during the last four weeks, in case labor should start.

WORKING

Again this is a matter of what you feel you can do and what your doctor advises, but there is no reason why any woman should not continue a mainly sedentary job until a week or so before delivery. Most of my women doctor friends, being fit and healthy, have worked until the last minute. One colleague was hurrying to an emergency when the waters broke and poured into her shoes. Off she went, squelching down the hospital corridor, tended the case, then set out for the labor ward.

SEX

The human female is one of the few mammals to permit sex during pregnancy. Contrary to folklore, intercourse can be enjoyed by husband and wife up to labor. Many women say that their sex lives have never been so good as when they are carrying babies.

SMOKING

The damaging effects of smoking on the baby, not just when it is developing (poor growth) but even after it is born (increased risk of infection and low resistance), are so well documented that every mother owes it to her baby to give up smoking during pregnancy.

GERMAN MEASLES (rubella)

The virus that causes German measles can pass from the mother's blood through the placenta to the baby. It is most dangerous in the first twelve weeks of pregnancy, when the chances of an abnormality occurring, such as heart defects and deafness, are five times higher than normal. However, the risk declines sharply after the twelfth week but by no means disappears. If you have not had German measles it is worth avoiding contact throughout pregnancy with an infected person or child. If you accidentally have contact with an infectious person go to your doctor immediately so that he can take a blood test to diagnose rubella and act promptly. If you see him within ten days of contact he may wish to give you an injection of gamma globulin to protect you and your baby. If you actually contract the infection, do not hesitate to consult your doctor, who will probably raise the question of abortion with you. Once you have had German measles you and your future babies are in no danger, so with an eye to the future try to ensure your daughters have it, or obtain vaccination against it, while they are young. Vaccination against rubella can also be given immediately after delivery to a woman who has been discovered never to have had German measles by a test done during her pregnancy.

16

VACCINATION

You should never have a *first* smallpox vaccination at any time during pregnancy, or a revaccination during the first four months.

DRUGS

Drugs can reach the baby by passing from the mother's bloodstream through the placenta to the baby, so it is a good rule of thumb not to take *any* medicines in the first twelve weeks of pregnancy, except under medical supervision. All new drugs coming on to the market must undergo testing in pregnant animals, and there are many medicines of all types that are known to be safe in pregnancy.

TEETH

Your teeth will not suffer at all as the result of being pregnant, though your gums may. During pregnancy the gums can become soft and pockets may form near the teeth, which will encourage infection. If this occurs the gums will be painful, tender to the touch and bleed easily. So it is worth seeking regular attention from your dentist. At five months the baby's milk teeth are forming, and it was thought that by taking only one fluoride tablet a day you could give your baby a strong set of teeth. It is now known that fluoride cannot cross the placental barrier to the baby.

DIET

Most women want to eat what is best for their baby and for themselves too. This is just as well, because the growing baby will take whatever it wants to the detriment of the mother. It is essential to eat some of the foods rich in protein, for example meat, fish, eggs, cheese or milk. It is not necessary to drink a pint of milk a day if you hate it, as long as you eat other dairy products like butter and cheese. Fresh fruit, vegetables and whole-wheat foodstuffs not only provide vitamins but roughage for the bowels as well. A pregnant woman should drink three to four pints of liquid a day, and water is best. Starchy, sugary foods should be eaten in small quantities. If you eat this kind of good, varied diet no vitamin or mineral supplements are necessary, with two important exceptions — iron and folic acid.

Anemia used to be so common in pregnancy it was considered normal. This is no longer the case, largely due to the fact that all women are given iron and one of the B vitamins, folic acid (often combined in one tablet), during pregnancy.

WARNING SIGNS

Though none of these signs necessarily heralds serious danger to you or your baby, if they occur at any time during pregnancy you should contact your doctor at once:

1. Bleeding from the vagina	5. Prolonged vomiting
2. Severe pain in the abdomen	6. Blurring of vision
3. A high temperature	7. The baby stops moving
4. Swelling of the hands or ankles	8. The waters break

Physical Changes

The statistics of pregnancy are quite staggering; here are a few:

1. The womb increases in volume 1000 times.
2. The womb increases in weight 30 times.
3. The individual muscle fibers of the womb increase in length 40 times.
4. The work done by the mother's heart increases by 50 percent.
5. The volume of the mother's blood increases by one-third.
6. The mother's kidneys filter 50 percent more blood than before.

The changes occurring in the baby are if anything more impressive, and in order to show how the mother and baby advance together through pregnancy I have drawn up a timetable (see p. 20) in which monthly progress is charted.

'Normal' Abnormalities of Pregnancy

DIGESTION

Nausea in early pregnancy is almost universal, is most common in the morning, but is by no means confined to that time, and usually disappears at around the third month. The exact cause of it is obscure, but there are at least two contributory factors, both related to

18

the high levels of estrogen and progesterone that are produced in a woman's body almost as soon as the embryo is implanted. First, one of the hormones, estrogen, can affect the stomach directly, producing a feeling of sickness; second, the levels of sugar in the blood fall and this brings on a feeling of nausea and faintness. Nausea is often precipitated by the sight or smell of food, and quite frequently by cigarette smoke, coffee and alcohol. Unless it is severe, there is no treatment other than taking a glass of milk and a cracker half an hour before getting up in the morning.

Vomiting is less common than nausea and usually comes on first thing in the morning. Again it is related to low blood sugar, and so the treatment is the same as for nausea. Most women suffering

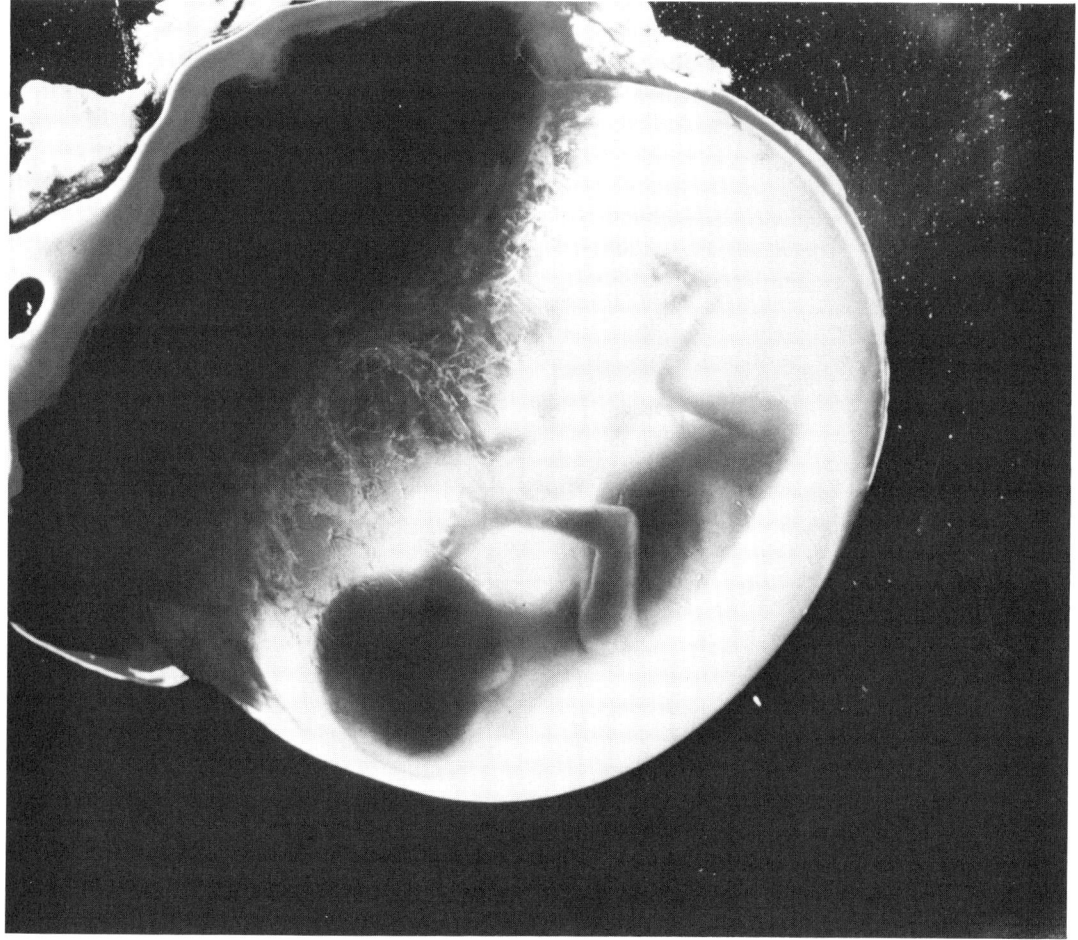

A fetus during the eleventh week of pregnancy

Pregnancy Month by Month

Month	BABY	
	Development	*Length and Weight (approx.)*
1	Heart is beating. Head, brain and spinal column have started to form. Limb 'buds' are forming.	
2	Embryo is still fish-like — eyes are prominent, mouth is recognizable and nostrils are present, but no external ears yet. Lungs are formed but are solid. Genital organs are developing and bones are forming.	Just over 1 in. (2.54 cm.) ½₀₀ lb. (25 g.)
3	Embryo is recognizably human. Face and limbs are fully formed with fingers and toes. Eyes have eyelids. Baby can be 'sexed.'	Nearly 3 in. (7.6 cm.) ⅛ lb. (26 g.)
4	Limbs and muscles in full working order. Joints can move. Fingers and toes fully formed with finger and toe-nails. Fine growth of hair (lanugo hair) all over body.	6 in. (15.2 cm.) ⅓ lb. (155 g.)
5	Eyebrows and eyelashes have appeared. Hair on head. Baby teeth form in jaw. Movement is very active. Fluid surrounding fetus increases so fetus can move freely.	10 in. (25.4 cm.) ¾ lb. (340 g.)
6	From now on baby can suck its thumb and cough and hiccup. Baby would survive for a short time if delivered. No fat has been laid down, so baby is very thin.	13 in. (31.8 cm.) 1¾ lb. (794 g.)
7	Baby is growing fast. Head is smaller in comparison with body. Fat is being laid down. Body covered in thick grease called vernix.	15 in. (38.1 cm.) 3 lb. (1.4 kg.)

Major signs	*Minor changes*	*size of womb*
First period is missed (amenorrhea). Breasts become tender and tingle. Need to pass urine more frequently than normal. Fatigue may be marked this early. Taste in mouth may alter — metallic.	Blood supply to all pelvic organs is increased. Sac left by fertilized ovum enlarges (corpus luteum of pregnancy) and produces pregnancy hormones which prevent further ovulation.	
Amenorrhea is established. Breasts enlarge and surface veins become visible. Nausea and sickness may be present not just in the morning. Still passing urine frequently.	Volume of circulating blood increases. Heart and kidneys begin to work harder.	
Nipple area becoming darker brown with tiny prominent bumps near nipple itself. Sickness persists. Weight gain may begin.	Wall of uterus is four times thicker than normal and begins to 'soften'; output from heart has increased by one-third.	
Movements may be felt from this time on, hardly discernible at first. Waistline starts to thicken. Womb is enlarging and pregnancy can be seen.	Uterus has trial runs of weak contractions that can be felt. From now on they become more and more frequent.	
Fluid (colostrum) can be expressed from breasts. Other parts of body may become pigmented, e.g. face, abdomen, inner sides of thighs. Palms of hands are pinker than normal.	Hair is affected by pregnancy: it may start to grow or maybe fall out.	
Skin of abdomen becomes thin and stretch marks may appear, especially if you are blond and if it is your first baby. Navel is flush with wall of abdomen. More weight gain.	Vagina and cervix enlarge in preparation to accommodate baby at birth. Pelvic bones and ligaments soften and loosen. Backache may be quite severe.	
Baby's movements are easily felt and seen. Indigestion and heartburn occur from now on.	Kidneys have reached their maximum output — 50 percent up from normal.	

	BABY	
Month	*Development*	*Length and Weight (approx.)*
8	Baby is perfectly formed and head is more in proportion with body. If delivered, eyes open spontaneously. More fat is laid down and baby has 90 percent chance of survival. Head faces down into mother's pelvis.	18 in. (45.7 cm.) 5 lb. (2.3 kg.)
9	Iris of the eye is blue. Nails have grown right to ends of fingers and toes and not beyond, and are very soft. Some hair on head is 1–2 in. (2.5–5 cm.) long. Lanugo hair is lost. Vernix is still present. Testes should have descended in a boy. With your first baby head goes into pelvis four weeks before delivery, with subsequent babies only one week before.	20 in. (50.8 cm.) 7 lb. (3.2 kg.)

from pregnancy sickness find hot, cooked food particularly repellent, so it's worth trying cold or uncooked food like hardboiled eggs, cheese, salad and fruit.

Heartburn is a painful hot sensation in the lower part of the chest under the breastbone, and comes on when the uterus is sufficiently enlarged to press on the stomach, that is in the latter half of pregnancy. To get relief you should take small, frequent meals, suck antacid tablets and sleep half sitting up against several pillows.

CONSTIPATION

This bothers many women during pregnancy and is due to the relaxing effect of the pregnancy hormones on the muscles of the bowels. It should not be necessary to do more than have bran at breakfast time or eat plenty of fruit and green vegetables or perhaps munch a few figs or prunes to alleviate it.

WEIGHT

'Eating for two' is quite unnecessary and undesirable, not only for your after-pregnancy figure but your health too. Though your appe-

Major signs	*Minor changes*	*size of womb*
Navel protrudes. You may notice ankles swelling at end of day. Ribs get pushed out by womb and this may be painful. You will feel very tired at end of day.	Volume of circulating blood is maximum. Level of progesterone is at its peak.	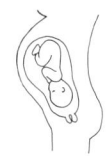
Breast growth is maximum and colostrum may leak spontaneously. 'Lightening' or engaging (baby's head going down into pelvis) is felt from 36 weeks onwards with first babies but usually later with subsequent babies, sometimes not until labor starts.	Wall of uterus becomes thin again and very soft. Different parts of baby can be felt. Lots of weak contractions may occur.	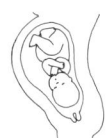

tite may increase there is no need to indulge it with fattening foods. Nibble on an apple or a piece of cheese, or keep some hardboiled eggs as a standby. Weight gain should not start much before the twelfth week and you will be rewarded if you can keep it below twenty pounds for the whole pregnancy. All weight over twenty pounds will remain after delivery, and worst of all it will be in places you hate, for instance on the shoulders and upper arms, the chest, tummy and thighs.

What accounts for the increase?
Weight of the baby — 7 lb. (3.2 kg.)
Weight of the placenta — 1½ lb. (681 g.)
Weight of amniotic fluid — 2 lb. (907 g.)
Weight of the uterus — 2 lb. (907 g.)
Increased weight of the breasts — 1½ lb. (681 g.)
Increase in blood — 4 lb. (1.8 kg.)
Total — 18 lb. (5.1 kg.)

When should your weight increase?
0–3 months 0
3–5 months 5 lb. (2.3 kg.)
5–7 months 10 lb. (4.6 kg.)
7–9 months 5 lb. (2.3 kg.)

The most difficult time to control your weight is between five and seven months, so a special effort is needed then by most of us.

HAIR

If you have dry hair it will probably get drier; if it is greasy it may get greasier. There is also a tendency for ends to split or break off and for hair to fall out, though this is most serious after pregnancy. Hair fall starts two or three months after the baby is born and goes on for anything up to a year. It can be so profuse that it can be really worrying. Now we know this hair loss is caused by the delayed effect of pregnancy hormones and is only temporary. About five months after delivery you can see new hair starting to sprout, but it takes about eighteen months for your hair to return to its former state. In the meanwhile treat it with care, using baby shampoo gently massaged into the hair *only once* and use plenty of conditioner afterwards. And avoid brushes — use one of those kind, wide-toothed combs instead.

SKIN

With the exception of the first couple of months when a few spots may appear on your face, the skin is usually in very good condition. Areas will become more pigmented and the darker your complexion the darker brown your skin will become. The nipples begin to darken in color around three months and about the same time a brown line, the linea nigra, develops down the center of the abdomen. Freckles and moles may turn a darker brown and occasionally brown patches may appear on the face (chloasma) in late pregnancy. None of these changes is permanent and will probably disappear within months of delivery, so should be left untreated.

Stretch marks can appear overnight and are due mainly to three things: an inelastic skin, the high level of progesterone that is reached during pregnancy and rapid weight gain. None of these can be controlled by rubbing oils on the skin or eating special diets, and all but a few stretch marks shrink shortly after delivery, so there is no need for pessimism. Really disfiguring stretch marks can be removed by plastic surgery.

BACKACHE

Low back pain is a common symptom throughout pregnancy. As mentioned before, progesterone produces relaxation of muscles; it also softens up ligaments, particularly those supporting the spine, so that the pelvis will give as the baby exits from the womb during labor. As a result the spine may be strained, especially if your posture is bad, but it is very rare for any permanent damage to be done.

VARICOSE VEINS

In common with the other muscles, the muscles of the veins relax during pregnancy to the point where 'blow outs' or varicosities occur in the form of varicose veins in the legs, or piles in the rectum. Piles may appear for the first time during pregnancy or existing piles may worsen, partly for the same reason as varicose veins and also because the growing baby presses on the veins in the pelvis causing back pressure to build up in the rectal veins with the formation of varicosities. Varicose veins and piles are rare in the first pregnancy. Varicose veins in pregnancy cannot be completely cured or prevented. They can be alleviated by avoiding excessive weight gain and wearing light supporting stockings or tights.

Prenatal Checkups

The statistics show that the earlier a woman goes to her doctor for her first prenatal visit, the higher the chance that she will have a normal pregnancy and a healthy baby. Good prenatal attention is the nearest thing we have to true preventive medicine, for tests can detect those mothers in whom complications may arise so that treatment can be given early enough. Prenatal supervision not only serves to check periodically that all is well with mother and baby, but also to remove some of the mystique from childbirth by encouraging prospective parents to attend classes on all aspects of pregnancy.

The first prenatal visit is the most detailed, with lots of questions about your medical history and your family's, your menstrual history and, if you have had babies before, your obstetric history. Personal details such as height, weight and shoe size (it gives a rough estimate of the size of your pelvis) will be taken; a specimen of your urine is tested for sugar and your blood pressure measured; your breasts, abdomen and heart will be examined, and a specimen of blood taken from a vein to find out your blood group and whether you are anemic and have had German measles. A vaginal examination may also be carried out.

Subsequent visits are routine — urine, blood pressure, abdomen, every four weeks up to twenty-eight weeks, then every two weeks to thirty-six weeks, then weekly until the onset of labor.

CARE OF THE BREASTS

At your first prenatal visit your doctor will probably talk to you about breast-feeding and examine your breasts, paying particular attention to the nipples, which should protrude to allow your baby to suck. If either of your nipples is turned inwards, at the sixth month you will be asked to wear a shell (a plastic cup with central holes to fit over the front of the breast) which gradually encourages the nipple to evert. At prenatal classes you will be encouraged to express colostrum at the fifth month by circular massaging movements, holding each breast between the thumbs and the fingers upwards to the nipple. A gentle squeeze on the outer part of the nipple area should express a few drops of the clear fluid called colostrum. The breast and hands should be smoothed with baby oil to make expression easy and comfortable.

Twins

Twinning is a characteristic inherited by both men and women from their parents, and it tends to skip a generation. Twins can be identical (when a single egg fertilized by a single sperm splits in two) or nonidentical (when two separate eggs have been fertilized by two different sperm and therefore can be different sexes). Nonidentical twins outnumber identical twins by about three to one. Identical twins develop within the same pregnancy sac and may or may not share one placenta. Nonidentical twins, on the other hand, are independent from the start and each has its own placenta.

The diagnosis of a twin pregnancy is sometimes difficult, and in 5 percent the second baby is not suspected until it is born. Clues are provided by a uterus that seems large for its dates and later by feeling two babies and hearing two fetal hearts beating. Twin pregnancies tend to be slightly shorter than single pregnancies, thirty-eight weeks instead of forty, though abortion is no more common. As there are two babies to support, the mother needs special care and great pains must be taken to see that she does not become anemic, that her blood pressure does not rise and that she does not put on too much weight (no more than 28 lb.=12.7 kg.); and she really does need plenty of rest.

Testing for Fetal Abnormalities

Amniocentesis is a fairly modern technique — a fine needle is passed painlessly into the pregnancy sac and a small amount of amniotic fluid is drawn off and sent for testing in a laboratory. It is rarely done before twelve weeks, but even as early as this it is possible to detect fetal abnormalities such as spina bifida and mongolism so that abortion can be considered. Later amniocentesis is performed to diagnose the severity of rhesus incompatibility and prematurity. Premature babies suffer more commonly from inadequate respiration than full-term babies. Amniocentesis therefore can be crucial to a baby who must be induced early, for it can be used to measure a baby's maturity by indicating the condition of its lungs.

Amniocentesis is not without its hazards, such as damage to the fetus or triggering off abortion, so it really is not justified for the purpose of sexing a baby, though it is possible to do so.

Clothing and Equipment

It is quite natural to want the best for your baby, but unless you have great self-control you nearly always end up being extravagant. Babies' needs are simple and few. Basically you need:

1. Diapers (cloth — two dozen, the T-shaped kind if you can afford them, because they are easier to manage — or waterproof disposable, which are equally good).
2. Four pairs of waterproof pants (for use with cloth diapers).
3. Four stretch suits (night is the same as day as far as a newborn baby is concerned, so there is no need for nighties).
4. Four undershirts.
5. Hat and coat for outdoor trips, possibly all in one if your baby will be born in the winter.
6. Two blankets of any description as long as they are warm; thermal blankets are best.

7. A crib or bassinet for the baby to sleep in, with two sheets.

8. A room that can be kept at a temperature of 18°C (65°F).

9. Feeding and sterilizing equipment (complete kits are available).

If you are breast-feeding that is all you require for the first few months. If you have opted for bottle feeding you should familiarize yourself with making up formula and sterilizing bottles. Immediately after bringing your new and hungry baby home from the hospital is not the best time to learn, as I found to my cost.

You can of course embellish your basic equipment as much as you like and there are one or two things I find indispensable, such as a waterproof pad to change the baby on and paper diaper liners to keep the diaper clean. If you want to keep all your baby's things together or if you travel a good deal, a plastic baby holdall with lots of pockets is very useful. Any clean, soft towel will do for your baby, but if you can afford to pamper him or her why not get one of those large, cozy, baby bath towels with a hood in one corner. The baby can be completely swaddled in it, impervious to drafts.

3 Labor and Birth

Nine months is a long preparation period for any major performance. During this time it will be impossible for you not to dwell occasionally on the difficulties you may encounter during labor, the pain you may experience and the possibility that your baby will not be entirely normal. Most of us are fearful of the unknown. Knowledge is the best antidote to the anxiety felt during pregnancy. Second and subsequent deliveries are nearly always easier than the first, and this must partly be due to the confidence that comes from knowing that if you could do it once you can do it again. So gather as much information as you can about pregnancy and labor; attend prenatal classes, ask questions of doctors and nurses, read books on the subject, and get your husband to join in, especially if he is going to be present at the birth. A new baby is quite an event for your other children too, if you have some. Make it a shared experience by showing them your enlarging tummy, letting them feel the baby kicking, and drawing pictures or following a chart of the baby's development month by month.

Having experienced childbirth with and without the presence of my husband, I'm in no doubt which I prefer. I found him a very great support; he gave me courage, he witnessed our son's first moment of life, which drew us close together, he was able to express his pride in my achievement, which added significantly to my pleasure, and he shared the first cuddles of our new baby. But of course it's a matter of personal preference. If you both want to be together for the birth, make sure you inform your doctor so that he can make appropriate arrangements. Most maternity departments are pleased to welcome fathers to the delivery room.

No one knows why labor actually starts, but we know that the baby almost certainly controls it. Just prior to the onset of labor, at a signal from the baby the placenta produces a hormone which sets labor in motion. The uterus responds by starting to contract regularly and with increasing force. Contrary to popular belief, babies do not have a predilection for being born at night; approximately the same number are born in any one hour of the twenty-four. The uterus is primed and ready for sudden action. All the way through pregnancy it has been having trial runs of weak, short-lived contractions that can be felt quite easily if you put your hand on your abdomen — the muscles go hard and tight. In fact many women experience these normal uterine contractions (the medical term is Braxton-Hicks contractions) intermittently during their reproductive years; they are most evident at the beginning of menstrual periods when they may be painful and cause dysmenorrhea (painful periods). However, once labor is fully established it becomes obvious that the largest and strongest muscle in your body means business; the contractions are strong and regular, usually fifteen or twenty minutes apart: they may be painful and they last forty seconds or longer.

Labor lasts six to twelve hours on average. With your first baby the average length of labor is twelve hours, though in 5 percent of women it lasts less than three hours, and in 10 percent of women more than twenty-four hours, but it is impossible to predict the exact length of labor. The delivery of second and subsequent babies is usually easier, smoother, less painful, quicker, calmer and less exhausting than the first, and on average lasts six hours. We even know roughly how many contractions it takes to deliver a baby: about 150 contractions are needed to expel your first baby; about 75 your second and third, and 50 your fourth and fifth.

Hospital or Home?

During the last few years there has been a movement away from having babies in the hospital and back to home confinements. Some circumstances, however, make hospital confinement desirable:

1. A first baby (you have not yet established if you have easy labors or difficult ones that require hospital facilities).
2. A first baby when you are over the age of thirty-five.
3. A history of difficult or complicated labor.
4. Twins or multiple births.

Even if you feel strongly about having your baby at home there are particular advantages to hospital confinement. Probably the only way to reduce the number of babies who die at birth is for doctors to be able to recognize those babies who are suffering from oxygen lack. For this they need the expensive monitoring equipment that is only available in a hospital. A compromise is to have your baby delivered in the hospital and return home within six hours of delivery.

Here are some of the advantages of home and hospital confinement:

HOME

1. You are with your husband and family.
2. You are in familiar surroundings.
3. You have a friend or relative to help — mothers can be invaluable at this time.
4. You do not worry about your absence from the family.
5. Your baby is always near to you.
6. You can do whatever you like with your baby at whatever time you choose (e.g. dim lights, quietness).
7. You can establish your usual domestic routine with your baby within a couple of days and he becomes a member of the family immediately.
8. You can have your own midwife to look after you.

HOSPITAL

1. There are skilled personnel ready for any emergency or complication.
2. You can be taught by nurses how to deal with the everyday care of your baby.
3. There is a pediatrician on hand to examine your baby and reassure you if you are concerned about anything.
4. You will meet other new mothers in your hospital ward.
5. You will be able to compare your baby to other newborn babies.
6. Troubles can be shared with other mothers, e.g. the discomfort from stitches, the difficulty in establishing breast-feeding, the pain of a cracked nipple.

Anesthetics and Natural Childbirth

Though labor need not be the painful experience many women expect, there are few labors that are entirely pain free. There is no doubt that fear, anxiety and ignorance contribute to pain. Finding out as much as you possibly can about what is happening to you and the baby during labor is one of the best ways to help relieve your labor pains when the time comes. If there is anything that puzzles you, or that you find difficult to understand, take the opportunity to clarify it with your doctor before you actually go into labor. This way you will feel relaxed and confident, the pain will almost certainly be less, and the pain that you do feel will be easier to bear.

I find most arguments in favor of suffering pain dubious. Suffering pain is not only unpleasant at the time, it is extremely debilitating and tiring, and even though you know you will have a brand-new baby at the end of it, it can be depressing. Having experienced both a painful and a painless labor, I am in no doubt which I prefer. However, there are many stoical women who for good reasons elect to have their babies 'naturally,' and that method is open to them.

Natural childbirth at its most literal means having your baby naturally, with you being fully conscious, able to experience labor and delivery, and in a state to take the initiative. It does not mean experiencing an unnecessarily long and painful childbirth, but being fully informed and prepared for what is likely to happen, so that fear and tension are avoided and you give yourself the best possible chance of 'enjoying' your pregnancy and labor.

Even if you eventually opt for, say, an epidural anesthetic, you can only benefit from attending prenatal classes on relaxation, the breathing techniques that help delivery, and instruction on the mechanics of childbirth. It also helps to establish understanding and trust between yourself and the doctors and nurses who will look after you.

For those who prefer some form of pain relief during labor, there is quite a selection to choose from, including anesthetics that are inhaled through a mask (like nitrous oxide), and analgesics normally given by injection (like pethidine). Anesthetics work by dulling our conscious appreciation of pain. As a result we lose our awareness of what is happening around us, and many women who want to experience every second of giving birth to a baby find this unacceptable. Before labor it is well worth discovering which types of pain relief are available in your hospital and, if possible, opting for the kind you prefer and telling the ward staff. You need feel no compunction to accept painkillers when offered if you don't wish to. It's your labor, so retain some initiative.

There are sedatives that relieve anxiety and make you feel calm and sleepy; there are hypnotics that actually send you to sleep, and there are analgesics that relieve pain without causing drowsiness. Once in the mother's bloodstream all these drugs pass across the placenta to the baby. A perfect answer would seem to be a painkiller that could be used locally to numb the pain of contractions, while leaving the baby untouched and the mother in complete control of her senses.

An epidural anesthetic fulfills all these criteria and in no way interferes with your awareness. It is aimed at anesthetizing the nerves that carry painful sensations from the uterus and birth canal to the brain, in very much the same way as the nerve from a tooth is anesthetized by a dentist. When labor becomes painful an experienced anesthetist can pass a needle through the lower part of the back into the epidural space (a space between the coverings of the spinal cord) and inject a sufficient quantity of anesthetic to deaden significantly the pain felt with each contraction but leave the level of consciousness unimpaired. A fine, delicate tube is left in the epidural space so that, if pain returns, which may happen after two or three hours, more anesthetic can be injected by your doctor without having to call the anesthetist. This method, which is available in some, not all, hospitals is practically 100 percent effective, though about five out of a hundred women continue to feel pain. Nevertheless they are in a better position to enjoy labor and be fresh and alert at the end of it. An epidural anesthetic can lead to a drop in blood pressure, which is rectified if you turn on your side. Very occasionally it is accompanied by a feeling of nausea or even vomiting, but this is transient and should disappear if you turn from your back to your side.

The Onset of Labor

There are three classic warning signs that labor is about to begin, though all of them may be preceded by backache in the lower part of the back for twenty-four hours or more. The first sign is powerful, regular, long contractions; the second is rupturing of the membranes, or 'breaking of the waters,' which is pretty unmistakable though not always a gush as many people expect — sometimes it is simply a slow leakage; the third is a 'show,' when you pass a small amount of bloodstained mucus — understandably this can be missed. When either of these latter two events occurs, telephone the hospital and tell them you are on your way.

First Stage

Labor is divided into three stages. The first stage is by far the longest and is measured from the onset of labor to full dilatation of the cervix. The purpose of uterine contractions during the first stage is to efface, or take up, the cervical canal. All through pregnancy, and indeed when you are not pregnant, the cervix is a fairly small tight tube a few inches long. As contractions become stronger, longer and more frequent, the cervix is stretched upwards and outwards round the baby's head. This is brought about by the strong muscles in the upper part of the uterus pulling on the relatively inelastic lower part which transmits the force of the contraction to the rigid cervix. Each time the muscle contracts, the cervix is stretched a little more. More important, it is held fast in that stretched position because of a unique quality of uterine muscle — it shortens its length each time it contracts, and is able to hold this length while still relaxing between contractions. Once the cervical canal has been taken up, the uterine contractions are directed toward dilating the cervical opening.

Dilatation begins slowly. The cervix has to open up to accommodate the widest measurement in a newborn baby's body, that is the diameter of its head, which is about four inches (ten centimeters), and this may take several hours. If your doctor examines you internally to check on progress, you may hear him say "she's three fingers" or "she's two inches," which means that your cervix has dilated to admit three fingers, or that he estimates the diameter of the cervix is two inches (five centimeters). As full dilatation approaches, only a small rim of the cervix is left. When this disappears the cervix has reached full dilatation and the doctor will certainly say, "She is fully" — fully dilated. This is the end of the first stage.

Second Stage

The second stage is from full dilatation to the delivery of the baby. Once the first stage is complete you will notice a change in the character of your contractions. They will come every one or two minutes and will last about one minute. In most women they become stronger and will be accompanied by an urgent desire to bear or push down. Many women automatically lift their knees up in an effort to make bearing down easier and more effective. Then, at the height of a contraction, a mother will quite spontaneously take a deep breath, hold it, and press downwards as though she wanted to open her bowels. Gradually the baby's head is pushed through the fully dilated cervix and begins to inch down the vagina.

During the last weeks of pregnancy the vagina has become extraordinarily elastic and can stretch quite easily to receive the baby. As the baby's head descends to the exit from the vagina you will feel it, and the desire to bear down becomes even greater. If you ask the doctor to hold a mirror you will see the top of the baby's head appearing through the vagina. This is called 'crowning.' The doctor may judge that the vagina will not stretch to allow the head and the rest of the baby through, in which case he will perform an episiotomy — a small cut — to make the opening bigger. This cut is made after some local anaesthetic is injected into the area, so it is quite a painless procedure. An episiotomy is done because a clean cut heals more easily and causes less damage than a jagged tear. After the placenta has come away the cut will be stitched up with sutures which dissolve away so there is no need to have them removed.

As the baby is being born he tilts his head upwards so that the first part to be delivered is the brow, followed by the nose and face, then the mouth and chin. At this point the doctor wipes the eyes, cleans the mouth and runs a finger round the baby's neck to make sure it is free of the umbilical cord. He will probably ask you to pant and not to bear down. At the next contraction, and with only a little effort on your part, the shoulders and the rest of the baby will slither out.

If you are not too tired, it is worth making the effort to sit up and see this actually happen. It is very thrilling to see your baby born. He or she will look bluish and be covered all over in a rather greasy white substance called vernix. The baby may also be a little smeared with blood, and his head may be a rather strange shape due to the 'molding' that takes place as the head comes through the birth canal. This is nothing to worry about — the head will go back to a normal shape within a very few days. You will notice that the face is

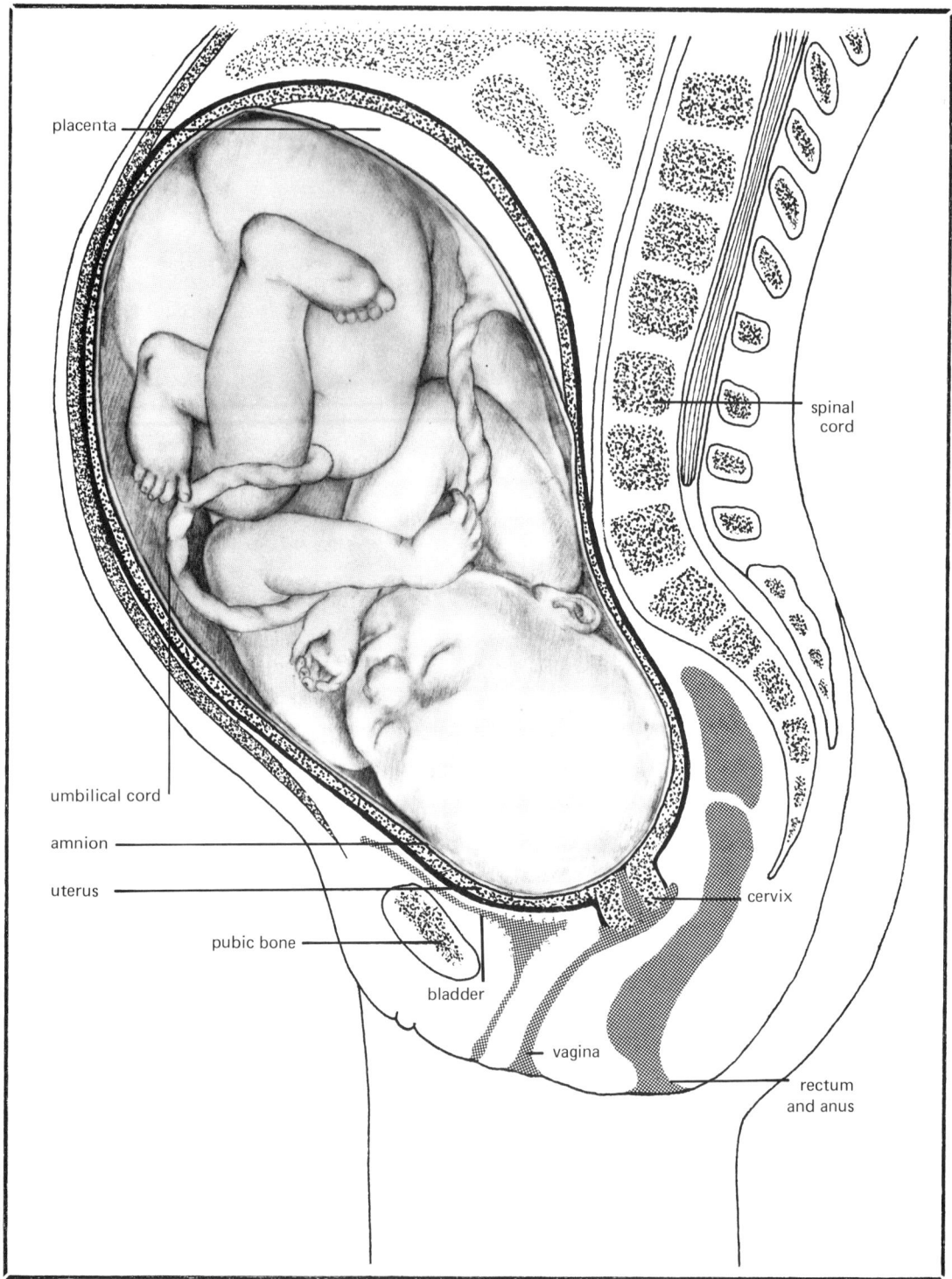

placenta

spinal
cord

umbilical cord

amnion

uterus

cervix

pubic bone

bladder

vagina

rectum
and anus

36

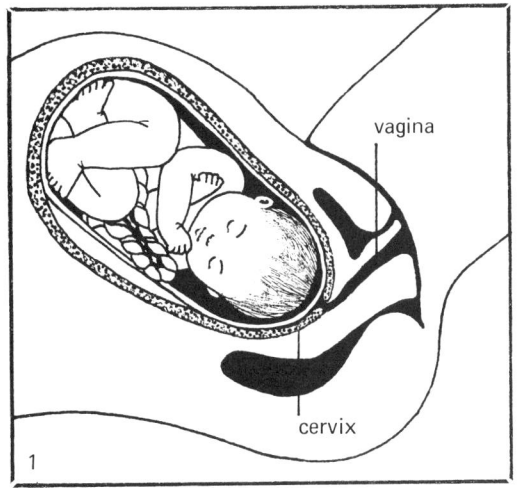

vagina

cervix

1

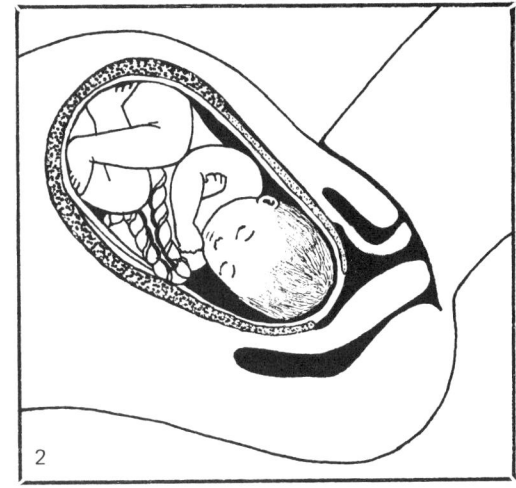

2

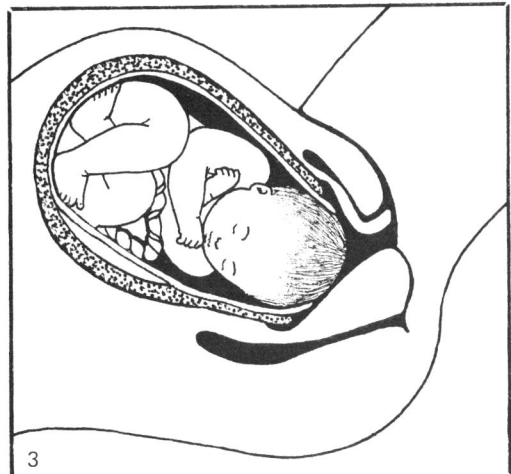

3

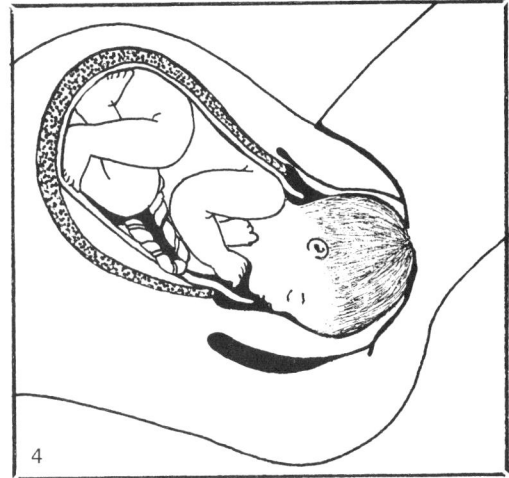

4

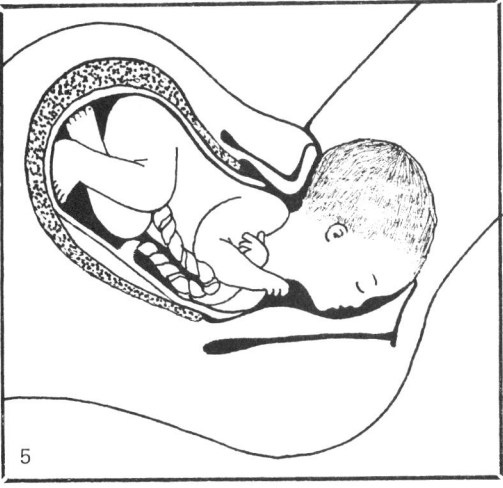

5

OPPOSITE The position of the baby within the uterus immediately prior to the mother going into labor. The cervix is a fairly small tight tube.

1 The cervix is being stretched upwards and outwards ('taken up') by strong, frequent contractions.
2 The rim of the cervix becomes very thin and then starts to widen.
3 Contractions are now directed toward fully dilating the opening.
4 Gradually the baby's head is pushed through the dilated cervix and along the vagina, which has become wide, short and soft, and the top of the baby's head appears ('crowning').
5 The baby's head is tilted upwards as it is born.

screwed up and he looks rather angry. The doctor will almost certainly put a small soft tube into the baby's mouth and suck out any mucus or liquid that has collected there. In a few seconds the baby will take his first breath, which will be followed by quite a strong cry, and at that point the doctor will clamp the umbilical cord. In one way this is a sad moment, because from now on the baby is no longer dependent on you — he is on his own. In a second the baby has ceased to be part of you, and after nine months it is both a sad and joyous parting. Very quickly after the first cry, babies become a healthy pink color. They stretch out their arms, their hands are tightly clenched into fists and their legs are slightly bent.

Most doctors will realize that the only thing you want to do is to hold your baby, and once the cord has been cut he will quickly be wrapped in a blanket just as he is, and placed in your arms. If the baby needs no further attention from nurses or doctors I think you should insist that you hold him or her right away. It has been well proven that it is very good for both of you if you do this. Besides the feeling of relief, joy, happiness, satisfaction and pride, some mothers feel other more basic emotions and I think you should succumb to all of them if you want to. Giving birth to a baby, after all, is one of the most fundamental things you will ever do, so if you feel like kissing him or licking him, or rocking him or crooning to him, or just laying him on your tummy and stroking him, do it as long as he's kept warm. Having come out of your body, being next to it is probably the most comforting sensation babies can feel, especially if they are next to your heart so that they can hear it beating. They have been hearing it for nine months and it will be very reassuring to go on hearing it for a little while longer. Any noise you make should be quiet, because newborn babies' hearing can be very acute and they are easily startled. Any movement should be slow but firm. The baby has been floating gently in a cushion of water for a long time and sudden movements make him fearful, especially if he feels he is falling. Though your request may not always be accommodated, ask if it is possible to keep lights dim. Up to now the baby has been in darkness.

Recently a French doctor, Leboyer, suggested that babies should be delivered in surroundings that as nearly as possible mimic those they have been enjoying in the uterus. He advocates semi-darkness, quietness, gentle handling of the newly born baby, and immediate possession by the mother. Once the baby's immediate needs have been attended to he may be placed on her abdomen and gently stroked. A sound recording of the human heartbeat helps the baby to familiarize himself with his new surroundings. Leboyer's practice is very appealing, but difficult to achieve in busy labor wards that are not readily prepared to accommodate such a radical change from established methods. It would be possible to follow Leboyer's suggestion at home, however.

We know that if a mother is allowed to hold her baby immediately after it is born, the third stage of labor, the expulsion of the placenta or afterbirth, is more readily completed. Some interesting observations have been made about the behavior of women toward their children according to how soon they were allowed to nurse their babies after delivery. It seems that if a mother is deprived of her new infant for longer than two hours after his birth she may be less likely to nurse him or make frequent physical contact with him, and when she does nurse her baby she may not hold him so that they can make face-to-face contact and look into each other's eyes. In later years she may be less loving and could be more likely to respond to misdemeanors with physical punishment rather than sympathetic discussion.

Third Stage

To ensure that the third stage is smooth and quick, the doctor will probably give you an injection of ergometrine when the baby's head is delivered. As a result the womb will contract again about four minutes after the baby is delivered. To help the expulsion of the placenta the doctor will pull gently on the umbilical cord, at the same time pressing your abdomen upwards and backwards. As the placenta enters the vagina you will again feel the desire to bear down, and the placenta will come away.

Forceps Delivery

Under certain conditions, such as delay in the second stage of labor, fetal distress, lack of oxygen which shows when the baby's heartbeat slows, or maternal distress such as the inability to bear down, forceps may be applied to your baby's head to help its delivery. This

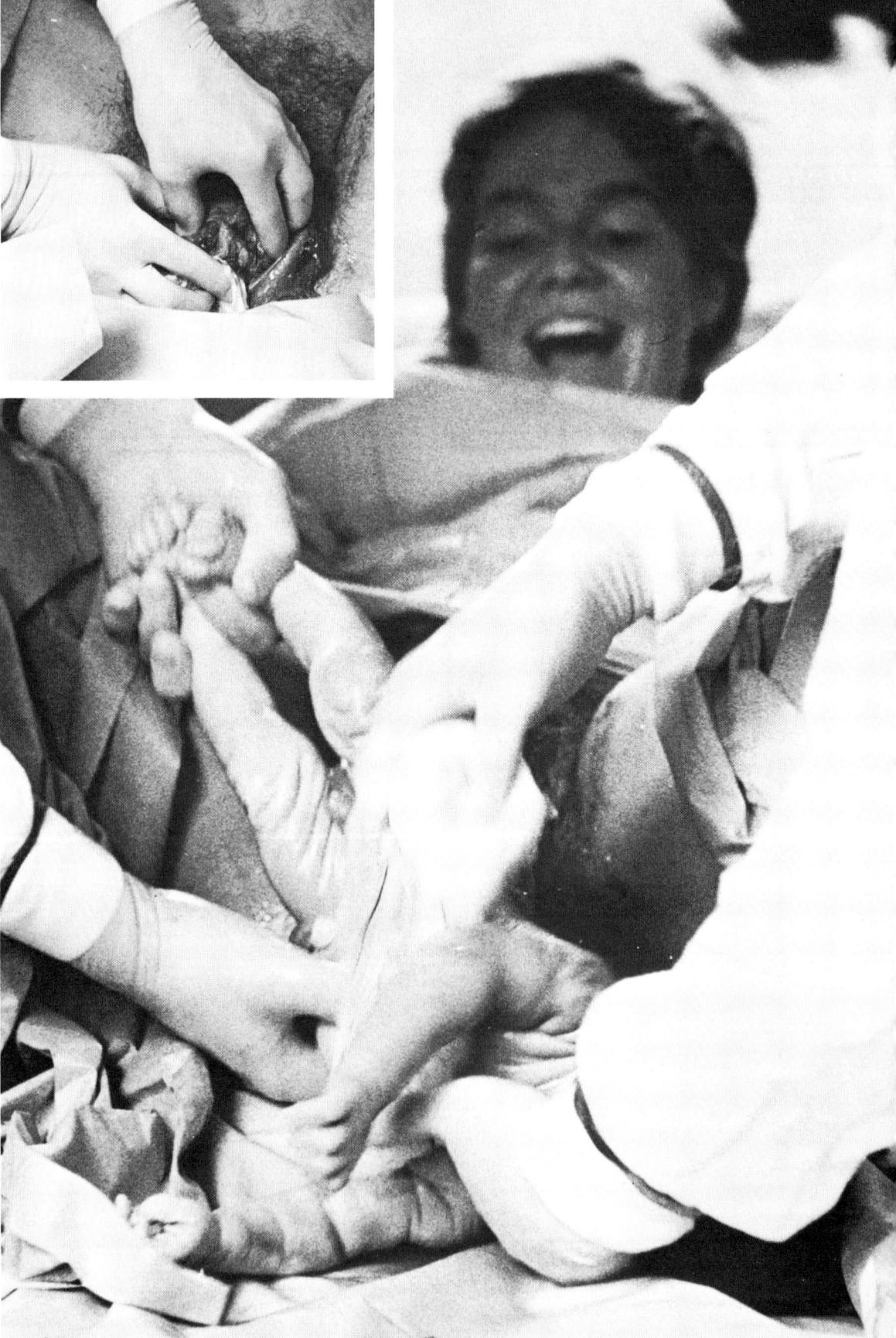

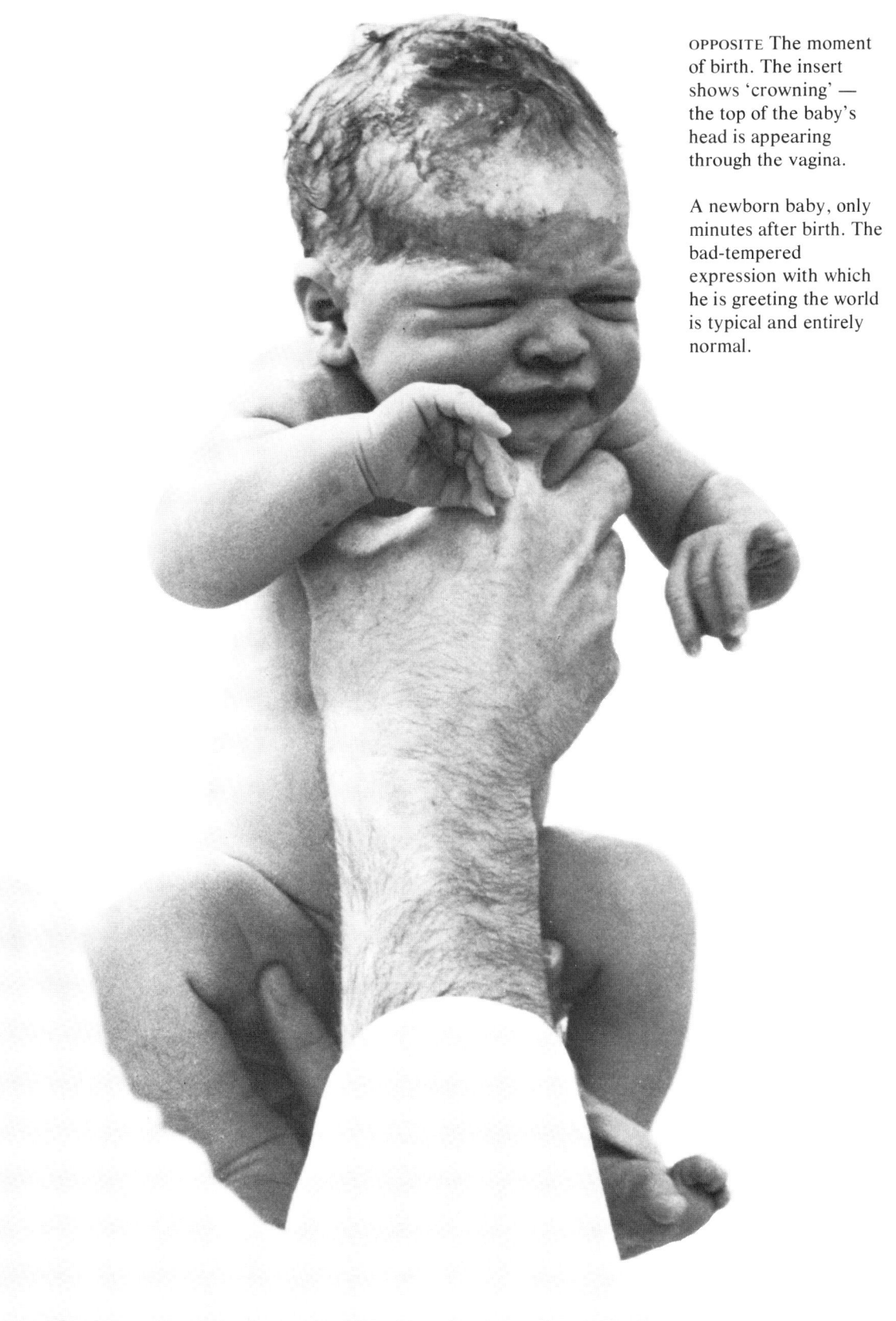

OPPOSITE The moment of birth. The insert shows 'crowning' — the top of the baby's head is appearing through the vagina.

A newborn baby, only minutes after birth. The bad-tempered expression with which he is greeting the world is typical and entirely normal.

is never done unless the cervix is fully dilatated and the head is right down in the pelvis and the membranes are ruptured. The decision to apply forceps will be explained to you and then you will be anesthetized so that it will not be painful. Forceps are made of metal with ends shaped to fit snugly round the baby's head without damage. When both blades are properly applied it is a quick and easy matter to pull the baby out gently. The worst that a baby suffers is a minor bruise or a mark where the blade was pressed to his skin.

Caesarean Section

Caesarian section is so called because it was included (lex caesarea) in Roman law in 715 B.C. as a means of saving a baby in the unfortunate event of its mother's death. The name also derives from the commonly held though improbable belief that Julius Caesar was delivered by Caesarian section.

This operation is performed in obstetrical units so often and safely now that it is regarded as a routine surgical procedure. It is considered when the baby appears to lack oxygen and speedy delivery is desirable; when the baby may be injured during his passage through the birth canal; and when mother and baby may be at risk due to prolongation of the first stage of labor.

As Caesarian section is a full surgical procedure, the mother is prepared for the operating room and given a general anesthetic, and the baby is delivered through an incision in the lower part of the uterine wall. Modern techniques mean that, everything else being normal, there is no reason why a mother who has had a Caesarian section should not have a subsequent normal delivery, though she will be advised to wait for a full year at least before becoming pregnant again.

Breech Birth

A breech baby is one that is born buttocks first. Most babies are in the breech position until about the thirty-second week of pregnancy when they turn upside down of their own accord. Four out of a hundred babies however, stay put. If your baby is one of these do not be concerned. Most breech labors are quite smooth and the babies quite normal. Your genital region may be slightly swollen but the swelling will subside in forty-eight hours.

Induced Birth

For one reason or another, your doctor may decide to induce your labor. This means starting it off artificially, usually by rupturing the membranes, and possibly initiating contractions by feeding oxytocin (a hormone which makes the uterus contract) through a drip into a vein in your arm. Induction can be carefully controlled so that the uterus contracts at a normal frequency and with normal strength. There is no reason why an induced labor should not proceed normally, be any longer than normal, be any more painful than normal, or not culminate in a perfectly normal delivery.

The reasons for inducing labor are medical and social. Medical conditions such as high blood pressure, rhesus incompatibility, and severe diabetes are a few of the conditions that are considered by obstetricians as possible reasons for induction.

Now that induction of labor is safe it is becoming more commonly used so that doctors and nurses can deliver their patients during the day, when they themselves are fresh and full hospital services and facilities are available to support them.

The First Few Weeks

Besides the happiness he or she brings, a new baby in the house, especially if it is your first, causes drastic changes of routine and demands adjustments that can be uncomfortable. It is foolish to think that everything will run smoothly, that there will be no crises, and that you will feel constantly overjoyed and happy. In the first place you will be surprised at how tired you feel; carrying the baby for nine months, especially for the last three, plus the exertion needed during labor, take a great toll of you. You may also find that your emotions are less easily controlled than usual. You may feel irritable, tearful and depressed. This is quite normal; your body suffers a considerable shock when the high levels of pregnancy hormones are suddenly switched off, and it can take a woman nine months to return to normal. Certainly your unstable mood will continue for at least a couple of weeks. Your new baby will in turn delight you, make you fearful of her small size and frailty and wear you down with her frequent waking during the night and crying spells.

It is as well to be prepared for a difficult first four weeks. If you observe your new baby carefully, you will learn what keeps her happy and, if you let the baby lead you, you will both establish a routine quickly. For instance, within forty-eight hours she will indicate to you the position in which she prefers to be comforted. Some babies like to be cradled, others like to be held upright over your shoulder. Some babies can tolerate a soiled diaper, but others are very sensitive to this and will cry as soon as they are wet or dirty and will not settle until they have been changed. And while most babies feed regularly every three or four hours, some enjoy drinks of boiled water in between feedings. It takes quite a lot of patience and attention to learn what keeps your baby happy.

Few babies sleep through the night before six weeks and all babies cry in the beginning. Most will cry once a day for anything up to an hour during the first two weeks of their lives, and very often you will not be able to find the reason why. I am afraid it is often a matter of nursing it out.

Daily Care of the Baby

Feeding the newborn baby is a subject on its own and is discussed in the next chapter.

It is good but not essential to bathe your baby every day. If it is to be an enjoyable, relaxed occasion, it is essential that you choose a convenient time when you can spend at least an hour with your baby uninterrupted. Most parents bathe their baby at the 10 A.M. or the 6 P.M. feeding. Much can be said for the evening, as bathing makes the baby feel drowsy and he is more likely to fall into a long, contented sleep. Once you have your baby undressed and in your arms ready for a bath, there is very little else you can do, and so you should prepare everything you need before you actually start.

You should make sure that the room is warm, at a temperature between 18 and 21°C (65 and 70°F). Have a warm towel ready for the baby, and see that clothes and diaper are prepared. Fill the bath with hand-warm water and put everything you are going to need on a small table close to you.

44

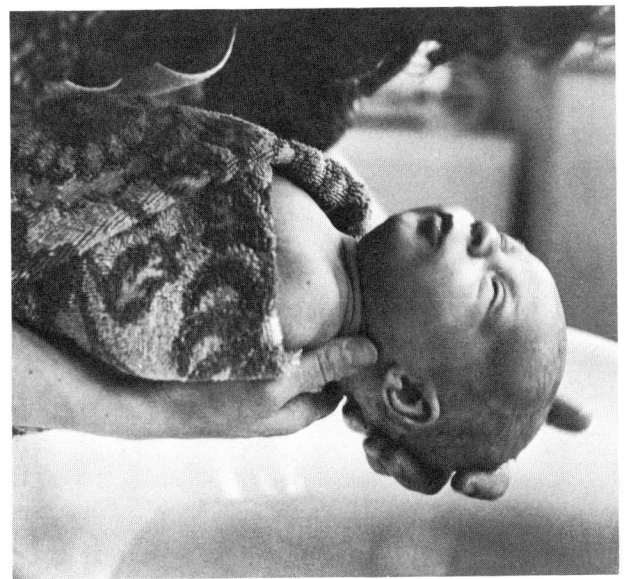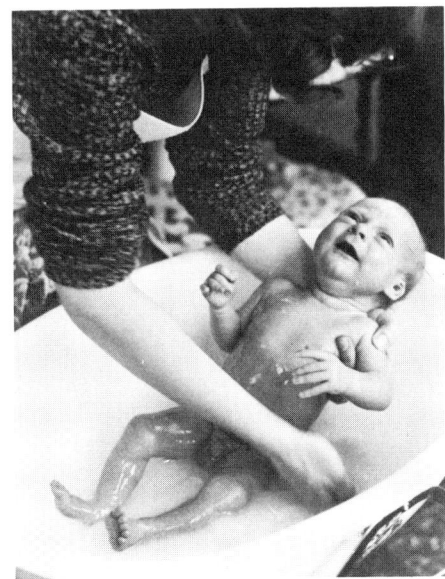

Wrapping the baby securely in a towel is the most practical and, for the baby, the most comfortable way of doing such things as washing his hair.

How to hold your baby in the bath to prevent slipping and make him feel safe.

Bath time is playtime, so make sure you are relaxed and un-rushed and you will both enjoy it. Routine in itself is not especially worthy but it does make things easier for you, so try establishing one. Start with the baby's head and face. Wrap his body firmly in a towel so that he is easy to hold, and then gently cradle the head in your hand and hold it over the bath. Take clean pieces of absorbent cotton, dip them in the water, squeeze them dry and use one to clean each eye and ear. With a washcloth, wash the hair and scalp. There is no need to use soap on any part of the baby's body, simply put a capful of infant cleansing lotion in the bath. Wash the rest of the baby's face with the washcloth and then pat head and face dry.

With your left arm around the baby's back holding his left arm, gently lower him into the water. Newborn babies seem frighteningly slippery, and a good tip is to put a diaper in the bottom of the bath, which will stop him sliding. Carefully and gently wash the whole of the baby's body, taking care with the skin creases around the neck, under the arms and in the thighs. Then lift the baby out of the bath, wrap him in the towel, and gently pat his skin dry. It is best not to

45

rub a baby's skin, as it is thin and fragile. If you dry very carefully in the skin creases there is no need to use talcum powder. I personally feel it is best avoided as it can dry up the skin and may become caked in the skin creases and cause irritation. In a few days the stump of the cord will dry up and gradually drop off; until it separates, clean the umbilicus with a little alcohol on absorbent cotton and then liberally apply a good soft baby cream (good does not mean expensive — plain old-fashioned zinc ointment is as good as anything) to the diaper area to prevent soreness and chafing. On days when you do not bathe the baby you can 'top and tail' him. This means simply cleaning eyes, face and ears, and the diaper area. At each change you can clean his bottom with baby lotion.

Newborn babies are awake for up to nine hours out of every twenty-four in the first few weeks, and you should make the most of them. Lift up, hold, nurse and caress your baby as often as you can. There is no doubt that it adds to the baby's security, and also adds to your satisfaction. Also, talk to your baby. Let him become familiar with your voice and he will soon be answering back. Long before your baby can see you, he will recognize you through your touch, your voice and your smell, especially your smell. Babies can smell their parent's presence in a room even when they are asleep. This subconscious recognition can wake them. They can distinguish the one who cares for them from all other people by the time they are three weeks old.

Looking After the Rest of the Family

Other members of the family, particularly children, may take the arrival of a new baby rather hard, so if possible they should visit their mother in the hospital and get used to seeing her and the baby together. It may help to preempt problems with very young children if you plan the entrance of the new baby rather carefully. When the family first meet you and their new sister or brother, make sure that your husband is carrying the baby so that you are free to give your attention to the other children. If you like, bring a present for them 'from the new baby.' Let them examine the new arrival; encourage them to fetch and carry at feeding and bath times, and let them know how grateful you are when they help you. Even quite a small child can safely hold the new baby if he or she is sitting down. Keep jealousy at a minimum by putting some time aside each day solely for your other children. Like any other mother animal you will be completely engrossed in your new baby and understandably many husbands feel excluded. All husbands should be capable of cooking a meal, cleaning up afterwards, and doing simple washing (if yours can't, teach him), but do make sure that he still has a share of your affection. He should be equally proud of the new baby and should want to help and to nurse the baby, especially when you are over-tired. It is just as important for the baby to get to know his father as his mother. It is only fair that your husband takes a share of getting up in the night, particularly at weekends when many men don't have to work the next day.

Looking After Mother

During the first few weeks after the baby is born it is very important that you get enough rest, and this means not only lying down for several hours each day, but also having a night of complete sleep now and again. If your husband cannot for whatever reason fill in for you, get a friend or relative to stay with you. Force yourself to do this, no matter how driven you feel to tend your baby.

You can start thinking about recovering your pre-pregnancy fig-ure by being careful with your diet, not eating starchy foods but concentrating on meat, fish, eggs, cheese, milk, fresh fruit and vege-tables, and by doing postnatal exercises. These are aimed at strengthening your back, tightening up your tummy muscles and toning up the muscles in the pelvic floor. Muscles regain their strength and tone if they are exercised often. It is simply no good to spend a few minutes once a day running quickly through a series of exercises and then forgetting them. It is much better to perform a few simple exercises as often as you can remember, say once every hour for the first week or so. Here is my routine:
1. For your back, put both your hands in the small of your back and arch backwards five or six times.
2. For your tummy, put your hands on your hips and pull your tummy in quickly and let it go again ten times.
3. For your pelvic floor, pull your vagina upwards in a movement that would stop the flow of urine if you were emptying your bladder. If necessary, actually do this to see how it feels, and repeat this

movement five or six times. Within a week you will be astonished at how much easier all these movements become, and how much fitter you feel.

If you are breast-feeding and develop a sore or cracked nipple, you can help it by keeping a pad of absorbent cotton soaked in baby lotion or smeared with baby cream inside your bra.

4 Feeding

Here are a few points to remember before I go on to write about feeding in detail. Whatever the method, the first principle of infant feeding is to feed the infant. There are no arguments against breast-feeding, but if you cannot breast-feed or have taken the decision not to, forget about it and concentrate on the needs of your baby.

Breast-feeding

Feeding is a subject of myth, drama, and dogma. You can get conflicting advice from almost anyone you speak to. Many mothers, prepared to do anything so that their babies will have the best, often soldier on with breast-feeding through a sense of duty, despite the pain of cracked nipples, engorged breasts, even the suspicion that their babies are underfed, until putting the baby on the breast can become a four-hourly nightmare. The trouble is that the more you feel you must breast-feed the more anxious you become, the more difficulty you have and the more inadequate and resentful you feel. The most important thing you can do is to be relaxed and philosophical about the whole business. And remember, your baby needs your care and love even more than your milk.

There are many reasons why breast-feeding is good for mother and baby. In the face of the mounting evidence in favor of it, let alone the natural urge to do it, it is difficult for me, as a doctor, not to be an advocate of breast-feeding. More and more people are coming round to this view and are resisting any pressures not to breast-feed. The most commonly advanced reason for breast-feeding is that it is 'natural,' and there are hardly any women who are not physically equipped to breast-feed. It is also natural to feel joy, pleasure, and pride that your baby is entirely supported and happy on food that is made by you. It is worth remembering that the pregnancy cycle does not finish with the birth of your baby but with the end of lactation. It is difficult to put into words the satisfaction that comes from knowing that you not only made a healthy baby but also that you are feeding a vigorous one. And it is probable that the physical nearness and pleasure helps to develop a close relationship between mother and baby.

Just as important as any of these considerations is that human breast milk is tailor-made for a human baby. We know for instance that it contains just the right amount of protein and minerals for the newborn baby.

As a medical student I was taught that the newborn kidney is relatively inefficient as compared to the adult organ. But this is only so in the context of an adult diet. The infant kidney is amply equipped to deal with a diet of mother's milk. However, the heavy sodium load in cow's milk can lead to a buildup of sodium in the baby's body and then to dehydration. It is possible that this is related to the increased number of crib deaths in babies fed on cow's milk. The protein in cow's milk is different from that in human milk and can cause an allergic reaction in a baby — the cow's milk proteins pass relatively easily through the baby's immature intestine and may cause eczema in some babies.

As long ago as 1948 a large survey showed that breast-fed babies were less liable to illness; there is less gastroenteritis, less chest infection, and less measles in breast-fed babies. Some of the mother's antibodies to bacterial and viral infections reach the baby before he is born, but *all* are present in the colostrum. In the first few days of life these probably exert a protective local effect in the intestine and may be absorbed straight into the baby's system unchanged to form an important part of the baby's protection against infections. If a mother has poliomyelitis antibodies it is not possible to infect her baby with poliomyelitis virus in the newborn period while she is breast-feeding him. Her antibodies in the baby's gut will kill the virus before it can do any harm. In addition to antibodies, there are substances in milk which can actually destroy bacteria, and while these substances are present in cow's milk a bottle-fed baby is not protected to the same extent as a breast-fed baby because they are inactivated if the milk is boiled.

Contrary to popular belief, breast-feeding is good for the figure. Recent research has shown that a woman sheds most of the fat she has laid down during pregnancy if she breast-feeds. She will probably have more difficulty returning to her pre-pregnancy weight if she does not feed her baby herself. Many women think that their breasts will lose their shape and firmness if they breast-feed. The changes that occur in the breasts are largely a consequence of becoming pregnant, not of producing milk. A hormone, oxytocin, is released during breast-feeding which encourages the uterus to return to its nonpregnant size and this hastens the return to normal of the pelvis and your waistline.

And all these advantages of breast-feeding are in addition to convenience, particularly at night; the milk being always at the right temperature; time saved not making bottles; money saved not buying equipment for bottle feeding; the baby suffering less from trapped air bubbles; the baby sleeping longer; even the regurgitated food smelling less unpleasant. And very important — rarely, if ever, do breast-fed babies become overweight.

There are, however, a few instances where breast-feeding is inadvisable. A baby with a cleft palate is very difficult to feed on the breast and it is as well to accept this from the start. Rarely, the mother's nipple may be so big that her small baby just cannot manage it. Occasionally a mother's health demands that she should not feed her baby. Your health is infinitely more important to your baby than your milk, and if there is any doubt do not breast-feed. A disease that takes the form of recurrent attacks such as asthma, or needs regular long-term medication, or that seriously weakens the body like kidney or heart disease, may cause too much of a strain to mother, baby and family to make breast-feeding advisable.

HOW TO START

For both mother and baby, the sooner you start the better. If you and your baby are healthy and you want to breast-feed, resist any delay suggested by hospital staff. Don't be put off by inflexible ward routine. Sadly it often seems that maternity wards are run for the convenience of the nursing staff rather than mothers and babies.

As a rule babies learn to take the breast most quickly in the first forty-eight hours, and have more difficulty the later you leave it. From birth onwards they are driven to feed by feeling the nipple in their mouths, and the earlier you take advantage of this natural urge the higher are your chances of success. If for some reason breast-feeding is delayed, most mothers begin to lose interest and by the fourth or fifth day the breasts may be so full and swollen that the baby has difficulty taking the breast. During the first few days moth-

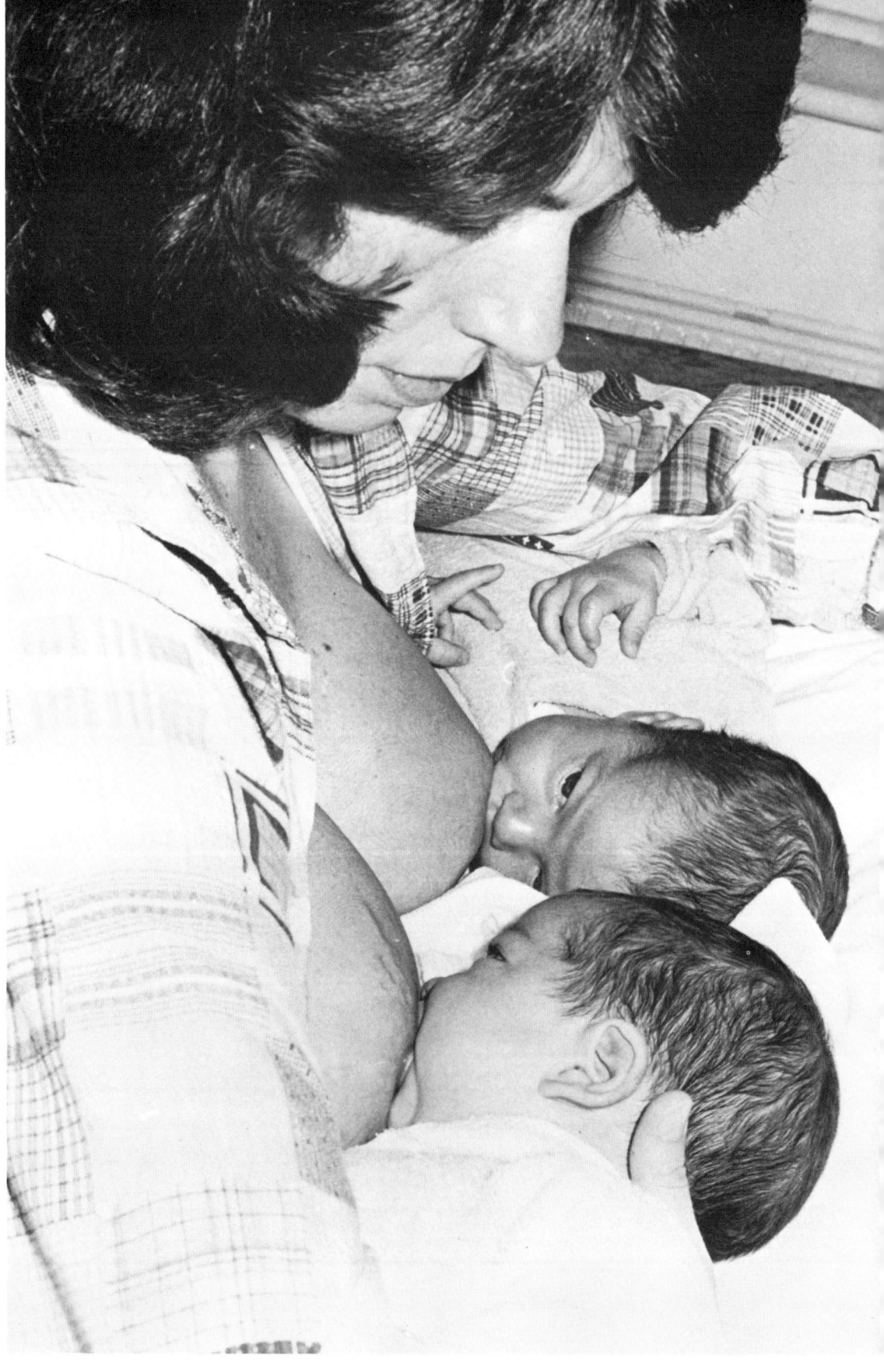

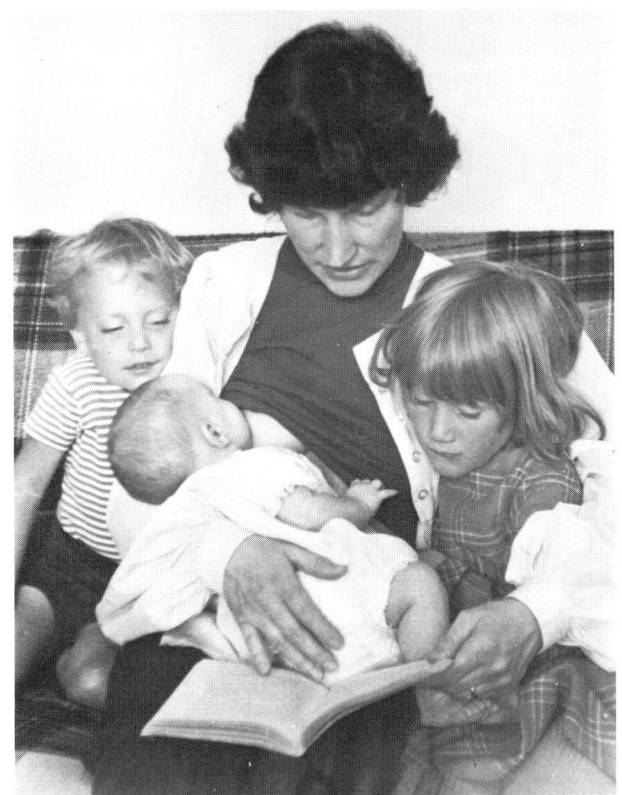
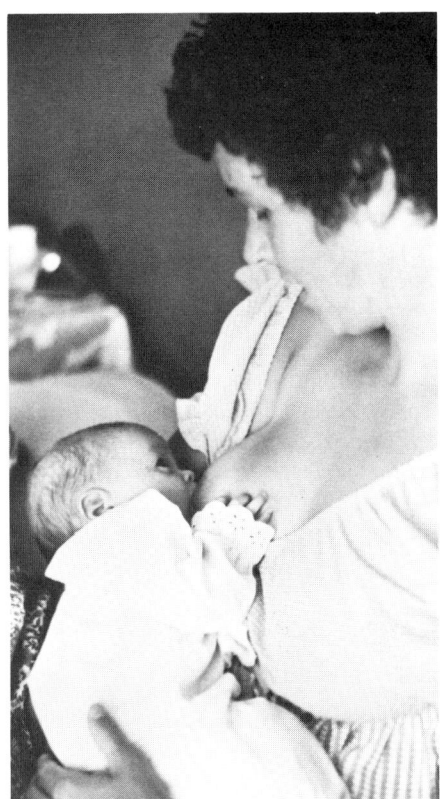

OPPOSITE Breast-feeding twins — so you think you've got problems with one!

ABOVE LEFT The whole family can join in with feeding.

ABOVE RIGHT Breast-feeding — it is important to try to maintain eye-to-eye contact between mother and baby.

ers are sometimes told that infrequent feeding will avoid sore nipples. This is wrong. If the baby takes small feedings often from each breast there is far less chance of soreness developing. Early, small, frequent feedings also encourage milk secretion and help to establish your milk-flow response to your baby's needs.

While we can think of breast-feeding as being natural, few of us have actually watched breast-feeding or had any instruction about it, so it is not surprising that it may be difficult to get started. The position of the baby and its head is important so that the nipple is accessible and the baby can swallow comfortably. The position of the mother is equally important, whether you choose to sit or lie —

53

if you lean back you are pulling against the baby and this can cause or aggravate breast discomfort. If you are sitting, make sure you are upright or leaning slightly forward. A cushion or a pillow on your lap can give you useful support. The baby should be cradled in your arm with back and shoulders supported and the head free. Try to aim the nipple at the baby's nose so that it will make contact with the roof of the baby's mouth, and make sure the chin is in firm contact with the breast. If your baby is held close to you she will usually lift her face and bring her mouth up to the nipple.

It is very relaxing to feed your baby lying down. It is best to be almost completely flat, with your body turned so that your nipple is about level with your baby's mouth as she lies in the crook of your arm with her back supported by your hand. Your baby gets most of her milk by the chomping movement of her jaws and tongue and the farther the nipple goes into her mouth the more efficient it is. Furthermore, if the nipple presses up against the roof of her mouth she is driven by instinct to feed. Taking a baby off the breast carefully can do much to prevent the breasts getting sore. If you gently but quickly press down on her chin you will normally find she lets go without a fuss. A special nursing bra (the cup can be freed to expose the breast) does away with the necessity of stripping for each feeding.

FEEDING ROUTINES

We are all accustomed to hearing and reading about three-hourly or four-hourly feeding routines. To my mind this implies inflexibility that is just unrealistic. Is there any reason why a baby should want food at a precise time any more than we do? It is far better to think of and carry out demand feeding. A new baby usually needs at least five feedings every twenty-four hours, and as long as your sleep is safeguarded you and your baby will be happier and get into your own rhythm more quickly if you feed him when he is hungry. As a general rule there is no need to wake a baby to feed him unless he has slept for a long time — say more than five hours. Gradually your baby's habits have to be fitted in to suit you and the family, and then there is no harm in waking him if a feeding is due and it is convenient for you to feed him. One of the kindest ways to waken a baby is simply to undo his blankets and free his arms and legs, and perhaps change his diaper. This usually stirs him enough to remind him he is hungry. If he is still full from his previous feeding he will probably fall asleep again and is best left undisturbed. If he falls contentedly asleep while on the breast the chances are he has taken all he wants. Breast-fed babies get most of their feeding in the first ten minutes and you can tell if your baby has taken sufficient because your breast will feel slack and empty.

AMOUNTS

If you are making plenty of milk your baby will almost always take as much as he needs. This does not mean he will take the magic figure of two-and-a-half ounces (70 grams) per one pound (450 grams) body weight per day. There is no definite amount that a baby should take at any age. The amount he needs is what makes him happy and gain weight steadily. Most babies get on surprisingly well with relatively little (less than ten ounces, or about 280 grams) in the first three or four days, and as your baby's needs increase you will probably keep pace with his appetite. Remember that your colostrum, which you produce in small quantities and which your baby only needs in small quantities, is very nutritious despite its thin appearance, and contains all the protein he requires. It is best not to think of each individual feeding in isolation, but in terms of how much your baby takes in twenty-four hours. Like ours, a baby's appetite varies, and a small feeding is nearly always compensated for by a large one later. Test weighting your baby after feedings is not a good idea unless he still seems hungry after an apparently good feeding and you need to know if he has had sufficient. Test weighting can make a mother feel unnecessarily anxious and inadequate. If your baby cries after a good feeding he probably wants a cuddle or just likes to go on sucking, in which case a pacifier should comfort him. Don't deny your baby a pacifier, as sucking is what he likes to do. Keep several in sterilizing solution ready for use. The chances are that he'll lose his pacifier and start sucking his thumb as soon as he starts to play with his fingers. By about the tenth day your baby should be taking (only as a rough guide) two-and-a-half ounces (70 grams) for every one pound (450 grams) of birth weight, and have regained the few ounces most babies lose in their first four or five days.

HOW LONG?

Advocates of breast-feeding say that two weeks on the breast is better than nothing, and from the point of view of giving your baby a flying start this is probably true. As a general rule, if you have a good supply of milk in the beginning you will probably continue for as long as you and your baby wish. However, when your milk starts to lessen there is no way of stopping it, and if you really want to breast-feed it is sensible to think in terms of three or four months.

While you're breast-feeding make sure your diet contains dairy products (a pint of milk a day if you like it), some first-class protein every day (meat, fish or eggs), and plenty to drink.

Bottle Feeding

There is no reason why a bottle-fed baby should not thrive, be as contented or gain weight as adequately as a breast-fed baby. In fact bottle-fed babies tend to gain weight too quickly. If you opt for this method and take pains to see that feeding is a time for loving communion with your baby, if you hold him close, look at him and talk to him, it can bring satisfaction, contentment and build up a close emotional tie between you. A bottle feeding should take about twenty minutes. A slow feeding will commonly make a baby irritable and tired. He will also swallow more air than he otherwise would. All this combines to make him unhappy and uncomfortable and he may refuse to finish his bottle. The result is a hungry, discontented baby who cries a good deal. One advantage of bottle feeding over breast-feeding is that both parents can do it. It not only serves to give the mother a much-needed break, but cements an early relationship between father and child.

SOME DOS AND DONTS

Do   1. Wash (with a bottle brush) and sterilize the bottle, nipple, cap, and screw-on top after each feeding (an easy method is the specially designed bath with sterilizing fluid added to water, which causes less wear and tear than boiling). Incidentally, once your baby is crawling it is pointless to go on sterilizing — simply keep all the equipment 'household' clean.
2. Buy lots of cheap nipples so that worn-out ones can be replaced.
3. A good routine is to prepare enough bottles for twenty-four hours in one go, filling each bottle with

prepared milk and keeping them in the refrigerator until needed.

4. Warm up the bottle just before the feeding. Standing the bottle in a jug of hot water is as good a way as any. Test the temperature of the formula on the back of your hand before you give it to your baby. It should feel neither hot nor cold.

5. Once your baby is fed, throw away any formula left over.

6. The nipple should simulate the human nipple as far as possible, so make sure it is soft and that the hole is large enough to let through an almost continuous stream of drops. Milk comes from the breast almost effortlessly when the breasts are full; make sure your baby does not have to struggle to get formula from a bottle.

7. Once you have chosen the brand of formula for your baby, try to stick to it. If she vomits a good deal or has running stool, consult your doctor. It is rarely the food that is to blame and in the early days it is better not to change brands.

8. Make your feedings exactly as directed by the manufacturers, mixing with boiled water that has been allowed to cool a little. Recently there has been a great deal of research into baby milks and the newest ones are very carefully balanced.

9. Babies who are bottle fed have more trouble with trapped air bubbles than breast-fed babies. In the early days you may have to stop halfway through the feeding to bubble your baby; as she gets older she will probably finish the whole bottle comfortably before she needs burping. To bubble your baby, sit her upright and support her with your hand. Sometimes this is enough, as air will rise and very soon after you hold her up the bubble will come. Occasionally gentle tapping or rubbing your baby's back will encourage her to burp. Bubbling, however, should not be viewed as a competition. If there are no results after five minutes or so, continue with the feeding.

10. Try to feed your baby in the sitting position as for breast-feeding.

11. Always put a little more formula in the bottle than you think she should be taking and let her feed until she is satisfied — it is almost impossible to overfeed a new baby.

12. Bottle-fed babies should be offered boiled water at least once a day.

Don't 1. Despite the temptation, don't leave a bottle heating on a warmer for the night feeding. Any bacteria that may be present in the formula or on the bottle can multiply if the bottle is left warming for a long time. If the formula is at room temperature it is quite acceptable to most babies.

2. Never reuse the remains of an old bottle.

3. Never add a scoop of powdered milk 'for the pot.' You may think you are helping your baby but in fact you are doing just the opposite. The young baby's kidney cannot cope with formula that is over-concentrated. If you are distracted while counting the scoops and forget the number, you should start again.

4. A baby should never be fed when she is lying flat on her back, as this makes swallowing difficult.

5. When making the feeding the scoop should not be heaped or compressed. A full scoop should be lifted out of the powder and any excess scraped off by running a clean knife across the top of the scoop, with the blade at right angles to the scoop.

6. Resist the urge to make your baby 'finish the bottle.' When she indicates she has had enough, do not try to force her to take more. If she needs more she will make it up. Doctors now feel that the model of a fat, bouncing baby is not what should be aimed for because fat babies may grow up into fat adults. If too much fat is accumulated in infancy, fat cells may be primed to take up fat for the rest of the child's life.

7. Never use undiluted, unboiled cow's milk in the first weeks of your baby's life.

8. Never leave your baby to feed herself unattended with a bottle propped on a pillow. She may swallow a lot of air; worse, she may choke, or gag on a mouthful and vomit.

Cutting Out the Right Feedings

All small warm-blooded animals, including human babies, need to feed fairly frequently. This is largely to provide fuel to keep their body temperature a normal 36.9°C (98.4°F), in other words to keep them warm. The less they weigh in proportion to their size the more often they have to feed. It follows that until an average-size baby of, say, seven pounds (3.2 kilograms) has substantially increased his weight in proportion to his size, he will almost certainly want to feed every three or four hours and is unlikely to drop his night feeding. As your baby puts on weight and acclimatizes to a day–night rhythm, you will probably find he sleeps longer between feedings during the night, but there is no hard and fast rule and you should let your baby guide you. By the time he is approaching ten pounds (4.5 kilograms) he will possibly sleep for five hours after the 10 P.M. feeding and gradually extend this to six. If he is sleeping soundly at ten o'clock leave him, and wake him just before you are going to bed so that you stand a better chance of having a good stretch of undisturbed sleep. Over the ensuing weeks he will probably take a feeding last thing at night, and wake between five and six in the early morning for his next one. This does not mean to say he will not stir! You can safely try to quieten him with a little drink (½–1 oz.=14–28 g.) of boiled water. Some babies get to this stage as early as six weeks, some take several months longer.

Adding to the Milk Diet

If you are breast-feeding there is no need to supplement your baby's diet with anything except vitamins in the first few months — mother's milk is short of vitamin D and a bit low on vitamin C. The best way to give your baby vitamins is in the form of specially prepared infant vitamin drops containing vitamins A, B, C and D, which are available at pediatric clinics and most good drugstores.

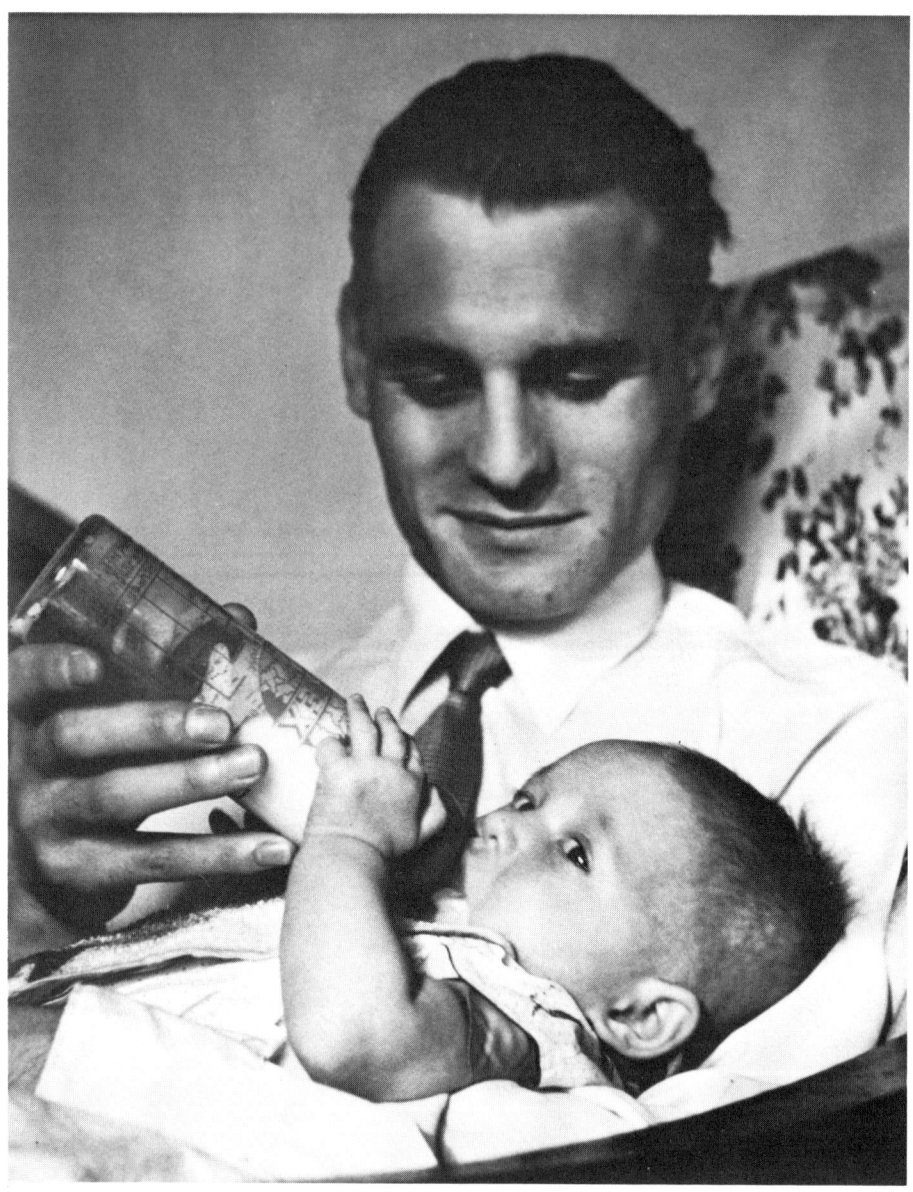

One advantage of bottle feeding is that father can feed baby.
Make sure you are comfortable if you are bottle feeding by
resting the baby on a cushioned arm and try to achieve eye-to-eye
contact.

They should be used exactly according to the manufacturer's instructions. Vitamin c can also be given to your baby in the form of
fresh squeezed orange juice diluted with boiled water (one part orange juice to three parts water). Most brands of prepared formulas
have vitamins and minerals like iron and calcium added to them in

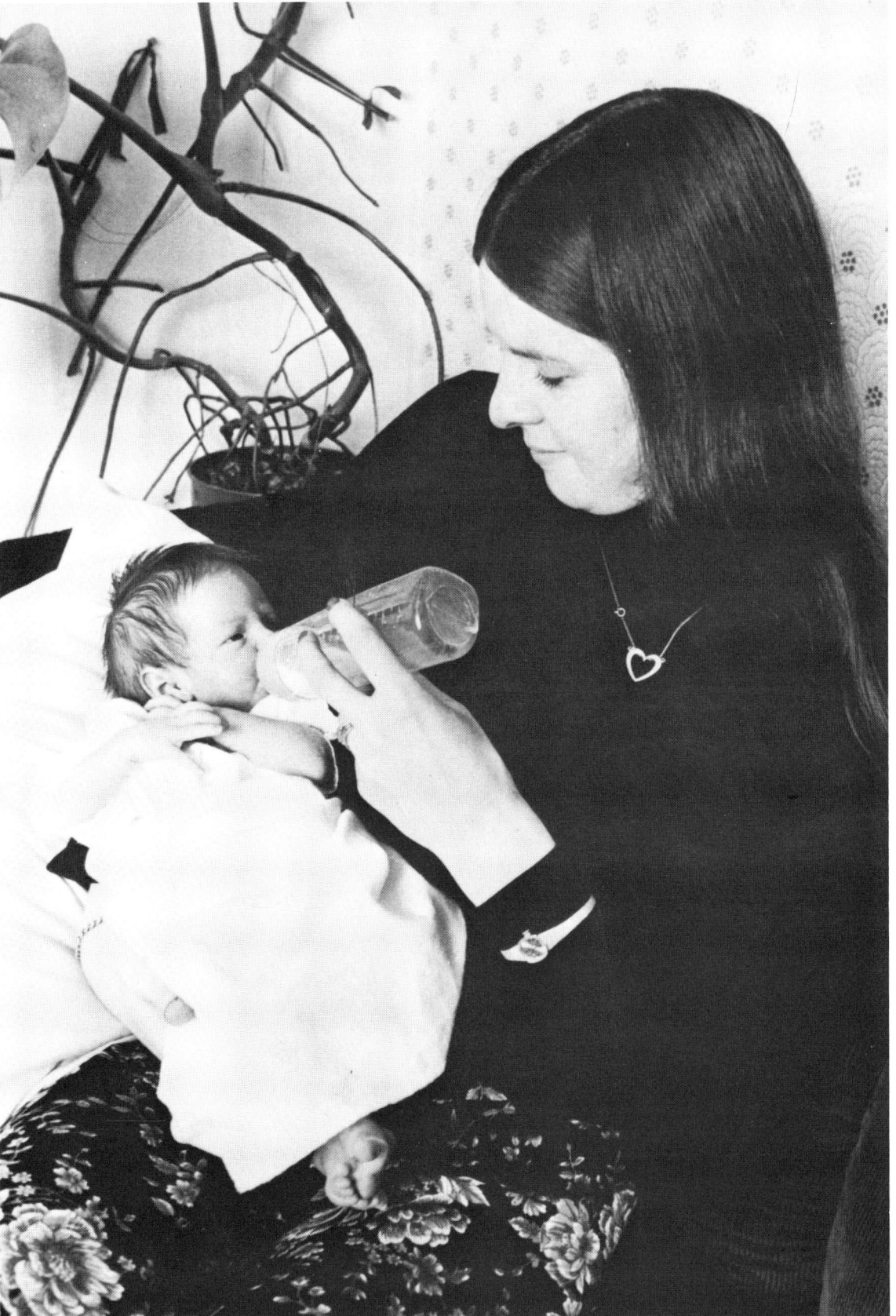

amounts that satisfy a developing baby's needs, so there is no real purpose served in adding to them. Fluoride supplements may be started from two weeks of age in areas where fluoride is not added to the water supply.

Up to the age of three to four months a milk diet (with the addition of vitamin drops in the case of the breast-fed baby or one taking fresh cow's milk or evaporated milk) fulfills a baby's requirements. At about this time however, the mineral content of all kinds of milk becomes inadequate for the baby's growing needs, and it is time to introduce variation to the diet if you have not already done so, though little is to be gained by starting earlier.

Start with slightly thickened mushy foods — a good one is baby cereal with protein and vitamins added, in small quantities only, say a couple of teaspoonfuls, and off a spoon if your baby will take it happily — perhaps just once a day until he is used to it. If he enjoys this, introduce a variety of other soft foods. Always make sure there are no lumps — your baby will not enjoy them since they may make swallowing difficult and even cause vomiting, and they pass straight through the gut unchanged. A few suggestions are strained baby foods, soft egg yolk or scrambled eggs, your own sieved stewed fruit or vegetables, minced meat or fish that the family are having with sauce or gravy and any milk pudding you cook. Remember that as soon as your baby is having any quantity of solid food he will need water as well to milk to drink. When he starts to cut teeth try crusts of bread or rusks — he will probably enjoy this sort of food and it can help to soothe tingling gums.

By about ten to twelve months your baby should be taking an adult range of food, though this can vary a great deal, but he should still take a pint of milk a day if possible until he is almost two years old. There is no hard and fast rule about the time to stop straining foods. Use your common sense and your baby's preference as a guide. If at six months he occasionally spits out a lump, continue with strained foods for a few weeks. Don't leave it too late, though, or he'll be slow to learn about chewing. Most babies are beginning to chew by six months or so.

It is never a good idea to force your child at mealtimes, either to eat or to use a spoon. A hungry child will eventually eat, and if bribed or told she can have dessert only if she finishes her first course, she will eat for the wrong reasons. Besides this, if you insist with a child against her wishes, mealtimes become a battle of wills and create a very unpleasant atmosphere, and may turn your child permanently off some foods. In the end the child will always win because there is no way you can make her eat. In no time at all the child will realize this and will no doubt use it eventually to get her own way. It is infinitely better to be dispassionate, especially as many children need less food than you can estimate. Some children thrive on only two meals a day — they are self-regulating and will eat what they need. A heaped-up plate more suited for an adult can intimidate a child. It is far better to give a child a small helping that she can easily manage and offer more when it is finished. You can of course encourage good habits — candies one at a time after meals (most children accept this: it is deprivation that makes them greedy and secretive); a supper of fruit and cheese instead of starchy cakes and cookies, but a cookie, say, midmorning. If a child goes through a phase (will not eat eggs or fish or spinach) it is best to play it down. She can get just as much goodness in other foods — there is nothing magical about spinach!

It's quite possible that as you introduce a new food to a young baby, say mashed banana, the stool will change consistency, color, smell and frequency. Unless the change lasts for more than twenty-four to forty-eight hours there is no need to take action, and don't exclude that particular food from the baby's diet forever. If you're worried, have a chat with your doctor.

Weight Gain

The rate at which a baby gains weight depends on several factors, including his birth weight and the size of his parents. As a general rule, new babies lose a little weight, large babies losing more than small ones, but the range is about four to seven ounces (110–200 grams). A full-term baby should recover his birth weight in ten days and subsequently puts on five to six ounces (140–170 grams) a week, so that roughly he has doubled his birth weight at six months and tripled it at one year. Many happy, healthy babies gain less than this. Weight gain is rarely steady, but a small gain one week is frequently made up by a larger gain the next. After the first year, a child's weight increases much more slowly — about seven pounds (3 kilograms) in the second year and five pounds (2.3 kilograms) in the third.

5 Crying

No one knows why babies cry. We know that certain things will make babies cry, and therefore know how to set about dealing with demands for comfort. But we do not know why their 'language' is in the form of crying. And a language it certainly is; most parents not only become attuned to their own baby's cry within a short time of its birth, but also soon learn to recognize a whole range of different cries and what each means. So for instance it is not too difficult to crack the code for hunger, pain, mild discomfort, irritation and bad temper. Between observant parent and child this dialogue can work quite well. One thing we do know is that a child who is nursed or held or is just in physical contact with its caregiver cries less than average — Eskimo and African babies who are slung on their mothers' backs rarely cry. This could well be because with their heads pressed close to their mother's chest or back they can clearly hear her heart beating, a sound they have listened to for most of their intrauterine life and that experiments have shown is a very comforting noise to a newborn baby. Or it may be that close physical contact, the smell of the mother and the sound of her voice, are all reassuring and obviate demands for comfort. The chances are that we in the western world nurse and hold our babies a good deal less than they would like.

A newborn baby can only be asleep, awake and quiet, or awake and crying. It is as well to expect a newborn baby to cry quite a lot — a few do not, in which case you will have an easier time than you expected, but very many do. If you expect it and treat it as normal you will not become anxious and you will find it a bit less difficult to cope with. To a newborn baby with a limited repertoire of communication crying is almost the only way of telling you something is wrong. If you remember that for six months or so the infant has been conscious of floating gently in the dark at a comfortable temperature with food always on tap, you can see that in the bright, hard, cold world there is a good deal of discomfort and quite a lot to cry about that does not necessarily constitute a serious danger.

Most babies need three or four weeks to acclimatize, to develop a routine, and to teach you some of their likes and dislikes; the frequency with which they cry after that usually diminishes. It is fairly easy to cope with a crying baby during the day when the chances are you are feeling strong and consequently sympathetic. It is quite another thing to have your night's sleep interrupted, and as few babies under six weeks sleep through the night it is probable that you will lose sleep trying to comfort your baby. I have learned that it is best in the early weeks to have the baby's crib right next to your bed so that at least you are spared having to trek, half asleep, possibly many times during the night to where your baby is sleeping. Many parents say that their babies have a particularly long crying spell — say up to an hour — once every day. For many this occurs in the early evening around 6 P.M., just before or after the evening meal. As with any crying spell, there is not necessarily any magic remedy. Most of the time it is a matter of nursing the baby through unhappiness.

One of the most difficult things for a parent to accept is that there does not always appear to be a cause for crying. Many quite understandably assume, 'If he's crying he's dying,' not to mention, 'If he's quiet he's dead.' But on countless occasions, after trying to pick up the message and attempting to exclude the common causes, you are forced to conclude that your baby just feels like a good cry.

Common Causes

What are the common causes? In the first few weeks it may be an air bubble in the stomach. Why are young babies so susceptible to this when we are not? Well, remember that for the first nine months they did not really use their digestive systems at all since food came to them in the blood — then suddenly within a few hours of birth they are miraculously swallowing and digesting. But the newborn stomach and intestine must get used to this new demand and it is not surprising that things do not always proceed smoothly. Young babies are particularly susceptible to swallowing air, and are sensitive to it in their stomachs. If the bubble is not brought up and passes down into the intestine, colic can result. This is due to sharp contractions of the intestinal muscles in an attempt to move the bubble on, with spasms of pain coming at intervals. It is recognizable when the baby draws his legs up sharply as each spasm comes. So it is worth being careful and conscientious about burping your baby. Occasionally colic can take a more severe form which is called 'three-month colic' because it just disappears at three months. Up to then it can be very distressing for parents and baby, as the baby may cry for long periods whenever he takes food. He can be helped by a muscle-relaxing medicine given just before his food. You must consult your doctor to obtain this medicine as it is available on prescription only.

Hunger is also a common cause of crying, and if your baby is crying for food it is natural to feed him. It is quite wrong to withhold a meal simply because it's not yet due. We do not always eat at regular intervals and neither does a baby. If a baby is ever left to cry for a long time he inevitably swallows air which causes him discomfort and prevents him from taking a full meal, but also he stands the chance of exhausting himself and he may be too tired to feed by the time you want him to. This does not mean you should feed him every time he cries. If he cries a short time after eating he may want you to nurse him — babies like company just as much as we do; or he may be thirsty, in which case he will enjoy a drink ($\frac{1}{2}$–1 oz. = 14–28 g.) of plain boiled water; or he may just like sucking, in which case a pacifier will comfort him. Do not feel hesitant about using a pacifier, particularly at night. His happiness and your sleep are more important than disapproving comments about pacifiers. If your baby does seem happy with one, buy several and keep them in a sterilizing solution so that there is always a clean one ready for use. And never leave home without one. Never put honey or any sweet substance on the pacifier, for it encourages a sweet tooth and contributes to tooth decay.

Many babies cry when they are tired and continue to do so for this reason until they are four or five years old. A tired baby can scream unremittingly and all your rhythmic nursing will be in vain. He will probably try to tell you by wriggling in your arms, and when he is a bit older by arching his back. All the baby wants is to be horizontal and still. Once laid down, with a little quiet talking or singing or gentle patting to calm them, babies will almost certainly quieten down and fall asleep.

Some babies seem not to notice a wet diaper, while others are fastidious from day one, and cry bitterly whenever they feel wet. What is more, they simply hate a soiled diaper and will cry until changed. If your baby is crying for longer than a few minutes, check and see that he is not wet or soiled, and change him if he is.

Dealing with the Problem

I often hear, "If she's clean and dry, burped and well fed, then she's all right, so let her cry"; or, "She needs to cry for an hour, it's the only exercise her lungs get." I could not agree less with this attitude. In my opinion a baby should *never* be left to cry. I have already mentioned that a crying baby may swallow air, so causing colic and making feeding difficult; also that she may become exhausted and irritable. Probably more important in the long run is that the baby very soon realizes that her pleas for attention go unheeded, that there is no loving human response when she asks for it. What can happen then is that she stops asking, and this may seriously damage her ability ever to form relationships with others. Her pattern of behavior, first with her mother and father, later with her family and friends, is almost certainly worked out in the first year of life. If friendship is denied her, a child may grow up to be introverted, withdrawn, shy of affectionate displays and repulsed by overtures of friendliness. This gives her a very unfair start in life. A baby really cannot be loved too much. It is wrong to believe that too much picking up or nursing will lead to a spoiled child. A child under one year cannot be 'spoiled' enough. She is in fact not being spoiled, but is learning about loving human behavior; and the model for this behavior that she will probably retain for the rest of her life is her early relationship with the person, or persons, who attend to her needs.

There is no doubt, however, that some babies are overdemanding — not greedy or selfish for their mother's attention, just more demanding than their mothers can bear without becoming resentful, fatigued and short-tempered. There are undoubtedly some occasions with all babies, even the placid ones, when a mother (and a good mother) would gladly do *anything* to stop her child crying and may momentarily contemplate doing it. So it is absolutely necessary for any mother, and particularly one with a child who is jealous of her attention, to arrange her life so that she gets time on her own away from the baby — and enough rest. One way or another, I think it is essential that every mother has at least one half day a week free to herself. Most people can accomplish this by getting a friend, or a relative, or a grandparent to come and baby-sit for a few hours on a regular basis. While most mothers, though dead tired, feel driven to tend to their babies at night, it is essential, if they wish to remain strong and even-tempered, to have two undisturbed nights and if possible two late mornings a week. As I mentioned in Chapter 3, husbands can usually do this night duty, but if this is not practical or possible it is best to try to get someone to come and stay for a few days with the precise job of giving the mother several nights of full sleep. In the first few weeks after delivery mothers really should rest for a few hours each day as well, and it is a good idea to plan in advance to have someone to stay who will make this possible.

The majority of babies respond to a routine, especially if it is established from day one. This doesn't imply inflexibility, more a rhythm that punctuates both the parent's and the baby's day. Ideally bedtime and everything associated with it should be happy. Most babies enjoy their bath, so you're off to a good start if you and she treat it as playtime when you can relax and she, hopefully, will get a little sleepy. Then supper and a drink, a story, a game, or a song, whichever works best, followed by bed and a firm but loving good-night *and leave your baby*. Some children as they get older develop preferences for particular songs that they like sung in sequence, or favorite stories that they follow in the book. Some will drop off to sleep listening to music, or while you sit by them quietly reading or singing.

If your child is ill she is quite likely to demand more of your time and attention at bedtime and will want to be nursed by you. And it's only right that you should respond to her demands. Unless you are prepared to accept this change permanently try to get back to your former routine as quickly as possible. Your baby will quickly learn that she can rely on your love when she needs it in the night, but coming into Mummy's bed after a nightmare for a quick cuddle, then back to her own bed, does not set a precedent.

Difficult Babies

There are, however, some babies (and more than people think) who do not settle easily and may pose great difficulties for their parents. One of our four sons is like this. The child who will not sleep at night is classically bright and intelligent, physically very active, interested in everything that is going on and openly affectionate. So while you may pay a penalty at night, these children are delightful and rewarding.

I feel there are a few guiding principles for coping with the sleepless baby. It must be said that the standard advice given in baby books just will not work. Be prepared for this and you will feel less frustrated and inadequate when the occasion arises. It's important to get your priorities right. No one — adult or child — can function properly for long without adequate sleep and parents are not a unique exception. Most baby books shy away from advice that seems to put the parents before the baby but in this instance I feel you must think of yourself as well. Sleep is the important thing, so to my mind you are justified in doing whatever is necessary to get it. There is nothing magical about bedrooms. Let your child sleep where he is most comfortable.

As a working mother I find it quite natural that my babies and I want to be together in the evenings; indeed I should be unhappy if we were closeted in different parts of the house. Because of my daytime absence, I feel very strongly that nighttime is my mothering time and so I'm prepared to be flexible about nighttime chores. For me, the sacrifices I have made in this respect have more than paid off. I feel we have found a special attachment because, importantly, I am the person who always comes to them in the dark. So if you find yourself with a child who is awake much of the night, do not be bullied by what you think you *ought* to do. Do what you *want* to do.

My youngest son is yet to allow us a complete night undisturbed so I have great sympathy for parents who have nocturnally wide-awake or demanding children. We are the kind of parents who get very distressed at hearing a child cry for any length of time (or knowing it even if we cannot hear it), so distressed that sleep is absolutely precluded. In any case we have never been able to let our baby cry for more than a few minutes because in that time he can become so upset that he vomits. So what solutions have we tried? How did we overcome the parents' dilemma of whom do you accommodate — yourselves or the baby?

The prompt goodnight after stories, games and songs never worked. What is more, our child did not stop crying after the fifteen or so minutes that many baby books suggest. We gave up putting him to bed and sitting beside him, sometimes for hours, sometimes in shifts, ages ago. Once we had decided to let him stay up with us until he was sleepy, however late, life became much easier for all of us. We would lay him contentedly on a couch in the room where we were spending the evening and at *our* bedtime we carried him to his bed. If he woke in the night we comforted him, gave him a drink and sang songs, but he did not always drop off again. We had to break all the baby book rules and take him into our bed from the time he was eight months old because that was the only way he would stop crying (and being sick) and we could not afford to go on losing sleep night after night.

He sleeps in a bed now but still wakes once or twice a night, so we have a mattress and a sleeping bag by his bed. We prefer to camp alongside rather than lose sleep sitting with him, returning to our bed, then having to get up if he wakes again later. My husband and I try to take turns and give each other a late morning at the weekend.

It sounds extreme. Few parents will find it necessary to do as we have done, but I know we are not unique, and some parents who have written to me are at their wits' end. Disciplinarians will disagree with our solutions, but the trite, simple solutions suggested by many just did not work for us. We have adjusted our night and sleeping habits to accommodate ourselves as well as our baby. Interrupted sleep has temporarily become a way of life, but suffering is minimized. While I know my son is demanding, I believe he is absolutely normal and I believe my behavior, while perhaps unusual, is also normal. It is an act of faith.

6 Illnesses and Minor Abnormalities in Newborn Babies

This chapter deals with newborn infants only. Common childhood illnesses are dealt with in Chapter 9.

Every mother, sooner rather than later, finds it irresistible to check over systematically every inch of her newborn baby, despite the fact that the infant has been pronounced fit and normal by the doctor. There are in fact few babies who escape without some minor and perfectly harmless feature such as a mole or birthmark. There are some variations of 'normal' that are so common they amount to peculiarities rather than abnormalities, and these are described below.

Shape of the Head

Your baby's head may not only seem large in proportion to the rest of her, but also appear to be a rather strange shape due to a swelling on one side. This is due to 'molding' that occurs as the baby passes through the birth canal. The bones of her skull are soft and pliable, and as her head is squeezed during birth they may even override one another so that her brain is protected. A swelling may form if pressure occurs in one spot for some time. In two or three days it will have disappeared. Swelling may be due to bruising outside the skull and while equally harmless, even if it feels quite hard at the edge, may take months to go. Incidentally, crumpled ears nearly always flatten out.

Breech babies may have bruises on the face and head but these signify no danger and will fade fast. If your baby's birth was aided with forceps, the marks may remain for a short time but should eventually disappear.

Fontanelle

Your baby's head continues to grow quite quickly after she's born, and to allow for this the skull bones on the top of the head are not fused together. This soft spot or fontanelle, which you may see or feel pulsating, is covered by a tough membrane and will come to no harm if you wash it thoroughly along with the rest of the head. Indeed failure to wash it will encourage 'cradle cap.' The fontanelle can vary greatly in size, and there are no standard dimensions.

Cradle Cap

This is due to the buildup of grease and scales of dead skin that cannot easily be rubbed off, as they are when they occur on exposed parts of the skin, because they are trapped by the hair. If they are left for any length of time the scales dry out and become hard and encrusted. They should never be removed with a convenient finger-nail, tempting though it may be, as this simply encourages the scalp to produce more scales. They should be gently massaged in the morning with absorbent cotton dipped in baby oil, and washed off with the nightly shampoo. It may be necessary to repeat this morning and evening treatment for several days to remove all the scales, but be slow and patient. Once the scalp is clear, keep an eye open for first signs of recurrence and apply the oil and shampoo treatment. This problem usually disappears by the time your baby is a year old but can go on longer. One of my sons had it until he was six years old.

Skin

A newborn baby's skin is quite immature compared with adult skin. You will no doubt notice that it can get very red indeed when hot, or mottled when it is exposed, or that the baby's fingers and toes go quite blue when the temperature drops. This is because the skin has not yet learned the trick of regulating the baby's body temperature as deftly as we have. This is why a baby needs to be in a fairly even temperature. The blood vessels in the skin are unstable and open up and close more readily than our own, producing sudden color changes. A baby's skin grows more quickly than an adult's, and as it grows from within, the dead cells on the surface are shed. Because a baby's skin is growing so quickly you may find the skin peeling, especially on the hands and the feet, and tiny shreds of skin in the folds under the chin or arms. This usually stops after the first four weeks.

Hair

Your baby may be born with a covering of fine downy hair (though many babies are born without eyebrows or eyelashes). This is lanugo hair that is normally shed during the last two weeks in the womb. Any remaining hair disappears soon after birth.

Birthmarks

There are a great variety of birthmarks from brownish freckles and moles, which are just collections of pigment-containing cells that have clustered in the skin, to larger pink or purplish marks that are due to increased numbers of tiny blood vessels or blood spaces (sacs through which the blood flows). Tiny red marks on your baby's eyelids or on the bridge of her nose or nape of her neck are often called storkbites because they are v-shaped. Most birthmarks of the blood-vessel type disappear in time, and even if they don't they are not usually noticeable. Some that look and feel like a strawberry (the strawberry naevus) are not strictly birthmarks but start as a red spot in the first few weeks and may get bigger before they get smaller. They seem redder if the baby cries or is hot, but by school age even large ones have nearly always shrunk and faded to a barely perceptible white streak. A mongolian spot is sometimes seen at the lower part of the back in children with dark skin. It is a grayish-blue stain in the skin, and usually disappears in the first few years.

One of the few birthmarks, fortunately rare, that does not disappear is the port-wine stain, and because of its vascular nature is not normally suitable for surgery. It is therefore necessary to fall back on camouflage with covering creams. Very good ones are now available in many shades to suit each skin.

Rashes

Because it takes several months for your baby's skin to stabilize, he may be subject to rashes which, reassuringly, go as fast as they come. The commonest is a red, blotchy, raised rash, possibly with small white bumps like nettle rash (urticaria). It is the most fleeting of all the rashes in a newborn baby; it may go in ten minutes or less, needs no treatment, and is nothing to worry about. Heat rash is a pinhead red rash that comes on the skin where the baby is hottest and sweats most, so it rarely appears on hands and feet. It is simply a result of the baby's being overheated; the treatment is to let him cool off.

As babies can't cope efficiently with temperature changes you have to change the temperature of their surroundings for them. Taking off a layer of clothing will help. One loose, thermal cover is better than two conventional tightly bound blankets. Never cover your baby in a waterproof or plastic coverlet that doesn't let the air get next to his body and the sweat evaporate.

Babies do get an assortment of rashes on the face. Most, if not all, newborn babies have tiny whitish pimples called milia over the bridge of the nose and cheeks. These are due to blockage of the oil and sweat glands and, since they disappear of their own accord, do not need treatment and should never be squeezed. When your baby is older, the introduction of new foods into his diet may produce pimples on his face. This doesn't mean he is allergic to each new food, he is simply registering the change in diet. Again, leave the spots alone and don't stop giving your baby the food. Both of my youngest sons developed face rashes at two weeks when they had their first fresh orange juice, but as they were well and happy I continued and the rashes faded and did not reappear.

Diaper Rash

Even the best cared for baby's bottom is susceptible to diaper rash. By changing often (at least with each feeding or when you detect a soiled diaper), and by cleansing rigorously with water and baby lotion, you may prevent it, but as a baby's skin is very fragile and the combined effects of urine and stool can liberate irritating ammonia, the skin can become broken and sore in a very short time, sometimes minutes. And, of course, some bottoms are more susceptible than others. Never leave a baby in a soiled diaper for a moment after you've discovered it.

Once the rash has appeared you must be extra careful about frequent changing and thorough cleansing (don't use antiseptics — they can be irritating to a young skin). Leave your baby uncovered with his bottom to the air for periods if you can and use a fairly heavy protective cream — plain zinc ointment is as good as any — when you put his diaper on. If you're not already using one, try a type of diaper that has a layer next to the skin which allows moisture to pass straight through so that the skin stays relatively dry. Some of the newest disposable diapers incorporate this in one and are also labor-saving, though of course you will have to weigh this against the extra cost.

Infections

If your baby ever gets a rash that is infected you should let your doctor see it and get the correct treatment. Don't use any old antiseptic cream that's lying about the house. Your baby's skin is delicate and you may only compound your problem and the doctor's.

Jaundice

As many as one in three healthy newborn babies develops jaundice, which lasts a few days, then disappears leaving them perfectly normal. The commonest type of jaundice is 'physiological' jaundice. This is caused by your new baby's relatively immature liver trying to cope for the first time (so far you have done it for your baby) with the routine job of converting the hemoglobin from redundant red blood cells into bile. This is sometimes too much for a young liver to manage, and temporarily the bile spills over into the blood and colors the skin yellow. The liver will soon get into the swing of things and physiological jaundice rarely lasts longer than ten days.

Jaundice due to rhesus incompatibility (you have a rhesus negative blood group and your baby has a rhesus positive one inherited from his father) occurs when a mother produces antibodies to her baby's blood corpuscles which can cross the placenta and destroy them. This may lead to anemia in the baby and jaundice after birth when the liver has to handle an excess of bile without the mother's help. About 15 percent of white women and 1 percent of black women are rhesus negative. A problem arises only when a rhesus negative mother is carrying a rhesus positive baby and hardly ever with the first pregnancy.

We now know how to keep a mother from making antibodies to her baby's blood. A simple injection of rhesus antibodies from another person will prevent the formation of antibodies against her own baby's cells. This technique promises to minimize the problem of rhesus disease. Routine prenatal tests for your rhesus blood group and the presence of antibodies throughout pregnancy prepare your doctor for any action that needs to be taken as you approach term or after your baby is born. It may be necessary to give your baby an exchange transfusion soon after birth to wash out all your antibodies, treat the anemia, and give the baby a fresh start. As it is impossible to change all the baby's blood the exchange transfusion may be repeated in the next day or so. The more premature a baby the more primitive his liver, and his jaundice may last longer than in a full-term infant. Rest assured that the amount of bile in his blood will be constantly monitored and treated promptly.

Eyes

SMALL HEMORRHAGES

A small crescent-shaped red spot may appear in the corners of the eyes. You may not see it until the baby is two or three days old, but a newborn baby's eyes are closed most of the time and it has probably been there since birth. It is a small hemorrhage caused by pressure on the neck or shoulders during labor, is harmless and will disappear in a couple of weeks.

SQUINTING

Until a new baby has learned to use his two eyes in unison (usually by eight weeks) he may squint. This is usual. If squinting persists after three months you should see an eye specialist; early treatment is important.

Newborn babies rarely shed tears — these usually appear at six or eight weeks. This is nothing to worry about; infants produce enough tears to keep their eyes healthy.

WATERING

If you notice persistent watering of one of your baby's eyes this could be due to blockage of the tiny duct, situated at the inner corner of the eyelid, that drains tears away down into the nose. Most blocked tear ducts open themselves before the age of six months, but if not will require a minor operation by an eye surgeon under a general anesthetic.

Snuffles, Sneezing, Breathing, Hiccups

Many things that a newborn baby does that cause us anxiety can be explained by the sudden change in way of life — from a dark world to a light one (that's why she may jump even in her sleep if you switch the light on), from a quiet world to a noisy one (she may flinch or cry at a loud noise), from a cushioned world to a comparatively hard, freely moving one (that's why she jerks her arms and cries if she's moved suddenly and thinks she will fall).

SNUFFLES

Some babies make a snuffling sound when they breathe through the nose; your baby may sound as though she has a cold, and her nose may even run a bit with clear fluid. This is partly because nose breathing is new to her and partly because she has small nasal passages. As she gets older and her nose gets larger the snuffling will stop and no treatment is needed unless breathing difficulty affects her feeding.

SNEEZING

Sneezing — and not just the odd one, but fits of sneezing — is quite common in young babies. This is because their noses are more sensitive than ours to any tickle and also because their eyes are very sensitive to light. This, surprisingly, can set off a sneeze (next time you want to sneeze look at the nearest bright light and you'll understand).

BREATHING

A baby's normal breathing pattern is different from ours; babies breathe faster and their breathing may look shallow. On other occasions the abdomen, which is normally protuberant, moves quite a lot as they breathe. This is because their lungs are smaller than ours in proportion to their size, and to compensate they have to breathe deeply and more often. When your baby is asleep you may notice she breathes quite deeply and quickly for a few seconds, then slowly, and then almost stops altogether. This is quite normal; her breathing will become stronger and more regular as she gets older.

HICCUPS

It is our diaphragm relaxing and contracting rhythmically that gives us our regular breathing. A new baby's diaphragm is 'irritable' and may give small jerky contractions. Each of these is a hiccup. Hiccups rarely if ever denote anything serious, and certainly not that a baby's food disagrees with her. Babies don't seem to mind them, so just ignore them.

Spitting, Vomiting, Stools

SPITTING

Spitting is regurgitation of a mouthful of food, during or at the end of a feeding. Some babies do it quite often, some not at all. It is never distressing to the baby, so keep your own distress about the smell to a minimum by having paper tissues handy or even under the baby's chin to mop up the overspill.

VOMITING

Some babies go a bit further and have a tendency to vomit from the very beginning. You can tell if vomiting is a sign of something serious by observing your baby carefully. If he doesn't seem upset, if he carries on as though nothing has happened, or smiles or just goes to sleep, don't worry about it at all. As he gets older your baby may actually seem to enjoy vomiting but, by way of compensation for the mess he makes, this sort of baby is nearly always bright and cheerful and cries very little. Despite your concern he will not starve and will thrive before your very eyes. My mother used to say "a healthy baby only vomits what he doesn't need," and that old wives' tale has been proven correct. Newborn babies need somewhat less than we adults estimate, and in the first few days or weeks we may give them too much too often — and they may derive so much pleasure from sucking that they take a bit extra. A baby rarely vomits a whole feeding. About two ounces (50 grams) of milk spread on the carpet can seem much more. He nearly always retains some and if he has gone short he will make it up in the next twenty-four hours. With a bottle-fed baby, check the hole in the nipple. If it is too large (too much too quickly) or too small (he probably sucks in air if he has to suck very hard), this may be the cause of vomiting.

When vomiting is serious, you as an observant parent will nearly always be able to tell. Your baby will probably *seem* ill — lifeless, whimpering, miserable. He may have spasms of obvious pain when he screams shrilly, or draws up his legs. He will probably refuse food. He may sleep a lot and not wish to be disturbed. He may strain when being sick and the vomit may project some distance. If he has diarrhea as well and vomits a large amount, more than once, call your doctor. Vomiting can lead to dehydration (the need for fluid) and it warrants prompt treatment. Vomiting in a small baby is a symptom of many sorts of illness, not just those of the stomach intestines, and so can herald a cold or ear infection, or a urine infection that on the face of it seems quite unconnected with the stomach. A baby with pyloric stenosis (the exit from the stomach is narrowed) does not appear ill until the condition is advanced. He does, however, look anxious, and is hungry immediately after being sick. Always seek medical help if the vomit is sour smelling, bile stained or blood flecked.

STOOL

A baby's first stool is greenish-black with hardly any smell, and he will pass it usually within the first twenty-four hours whether he has been fed or not. Over the next three to four days the stools become light brownish-yellow (with a texture like scrambled eggs). The stools of a breast-fed baby are always soft, and usually yellow with occasional green patches. A totally green stool is perfectly normal. It means that the bile system is beginning to work and that that particular feeding passed quickly through the intestine. The stools of a bottle-fed baby are firmer, browner and smellier. In the first few days your baby may pass a small stool with every meal, which is also quite normal. Within the next few weeks the stools will become less frequent, perhaps one a day or one every few days. There is so little waste from breast milk that one stool every seven days is no cause for alarm in a breast-fed baby. Constipation does not occur in babies who are purely breast-fed. Looseness in itself need not worry you, nor need a little mucus. On the other hand, watery stools, especially if your baby has lost his appetite and seems ill, warrant contacting your doctor. With a bottle-fed baby there is more waste and he should pass a stool every day. Missing the odd day is normal but if the stools are persistently hard and infrequent try adding a little more sugar to the next day's food to loosen him up. In the summertime he may be sweating a good deal and his body will conserve water by drying out his stool, so small drinks of boiled water or diluted orange juice between meals can help. If your baby is thirsty after eating, try making up his milk with an extra ounce or two of water to the normal number of scoops of powder.

Other Causes of Worry

EPITHELIAL PEARLS

These are two white spots normally on either side of a baby's hard palate (the roof of the mouth). They are rarely seen, largely because one doesn't look, but if you do see them don't worry — they should be there. They may also occur on the penis.

BREAST ENGORGEMENT

Babies of both sexes may be born with enlarged breasts, quite hard to the touch. This is because the high level of pregnancy hormones in your body can reach your baby across the placenta. The breasts gradually shrink in the ensuing weeks.

VAGINAL DISCHARGE

For the same reason as above, a baby girl may pass a little reddish discharge from the vagina, normally between the third and seventh day.

CORD WON'T SEPARATE

Keep the cord dry, so that it separates slowly. Most cords separate by three weeks.

FAILURE TO STRAIGHTEN THE LEGS

Babies have been in a fairly tightly curled-up ball for some months and for the first ten days or so are loath to stretch out. Indeed at first they can't — they need time to unwind!

HERNIAS

You may notice that a small bulge appears around your baby's umbilicus when he coughs or cries. This is due to a small split in the muscles of the abdomen. He will come to no harm and it will almost certainly close up before he is six months old. You may also notice a hernia in the region of his scrotum. Draw your doctor's attention to it immediately as it may need treatment later. To most mothers the opening in the skin over the end of the penis appears to be far too small to be normal, but as the pediatrician said to me when I queried this with my first baby, "What appears to be smaller at birth than nature intended becomes large enough to cover most contingencies in later years." Seek assurance from your doctor if you are worried.

TONGUE-TIE

A small degree of tongue-tie (the underside of the tongue is tethered to the floor of the mouth) is so common as to be considered normal in every newborn baby, and rarely interferes with sucking or speech development. If you are worried, draw it to the attention of your doctor.

NAILS

Babies' nails grow very quickly. Keep them regularly trimmed, particularly if your baby is scratching herself.

SUCKING BLISTERS

My youngest son was born with large blisters on top of his wrists and forearms. Even the nurse couldn't explain them. The explanation became obvious within a few hours of his birth, when he clamped his wrists in his mouth and sucked fiercely. He had been sucking his wrists while still in my womb. He stopped trying to do this as feeding became established and the blisters dried up without treatment; they were simply kept clean and dry.

THRUSH

This is caused by a fungus called Candida albicans, which normally lives in small numbers in our intestines. It may multiply to cause an infection, affecting newborn babies mainly in the mouth where it appears as white patches on the cheeks, tongue and palate. It can resemble milk curd, but can be distinguished because it does not wipe off easily. It may make your baby's mouth sore enough to refuse food. It is normally treated with drops that can be obtained on prescription. Candida may complicate diaper rash and you will need special cream from your doctor to eradicate it from the skin.

7 Physical and Mental Development

It's very tempting to try to chart a baby's progress and to state the precise size and weight she should have reached, the number of teeth that should have erupted, the skills and understanding she should have acquired at any given age. In other words, to pigeon-hole and categorize her. This is very undesirable. To a mother who is not aware of the wide range of the normal, it can be frightening if she thinks her baby is not developing as she should, or is falling behind. What is more, it is not medically possible to be absolutely precise, and if precision is attempted it can lead to dangerous oversimplification.

How to Measure Development

Normality, as far as a growing baby or child is concerned, is something that few doctors would attempt to define. A child can be very much below the average weight for her age, for example, but still be the normal weight for *herself*. Normality should properly be assessed by comparison with what has previously affected that particular baby and not with what other babies of a similar age are doing. A baby's progress depends on many interrelated factors. Weight, for instance, is affected by the size of the parents, by birth weight, and by how the baby has been fed. And so it's much better to judge weight by the baby's record over the months, rather than by taking a single measurement. Furthermore, no two babies grow at the same rate.

An 'average' is the most accurate measurement that a doctor can come up with and at best it is imperfect, for many normal, healthy children deviate greatly from the average. The average child is only a theoretical consideration, a composite of the fastest-growing and slowest-growing children, of the best-fed with the poorest-fed children, of the happiest with the unhappiest children. The 'average' is the middle of the normal range; the range itself may spread a long way up or down from the average, but on its own the average gives no indication of this spread. So it's dangerous to compare your child with what is considered average. And while we say that on average a child should have doubled her birth weight at six months and trebled it at a year, we must remember this is only true for the child of *average* birth weight.

Scientists have devised a way of expressing measurement to take some account of the usual spread from the average. It's called the 'percentile' system and tells you how often any particular measurement occurs in one hundred other children. The fortieth percentile means that in 40 percent of children studied the measurement we're interested in fell below that figure. It follows that 90 percent of all measurements taken will fall between the fifth and ninety-fifth percentiles. When my last son was born at a weight of just under six pounds eight ounces (3 kilograms), the obstetrician said his weight was in the tenth percentile, which meant that only ten percent of children were born weighing less than him — he was quite a low birth weight baby. Using percentile charts it's possible to compare measurements of a single child with those of other children. It's probably the fairest and most realistic way of drawing comparisons. This is the sort of chart that's used.

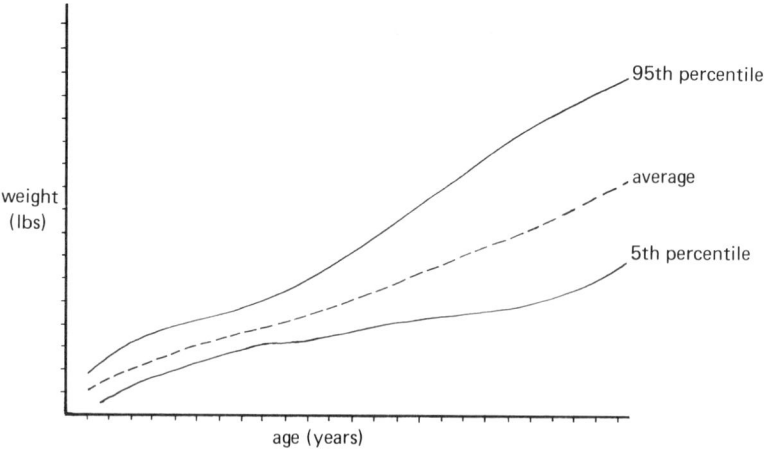

There are certain axioms that apply to development in all children:

1. Though development may slow down and speed up it is continuous, and the child can make progress not only in what he does but in how he does it.
2. A child can only develop as fast as the brain and nervous system are developing. The parts of the brain associated with a skill like walking must be mature before walking can be learned.
3. Though the *rate* of development may vary, the *sequence* of development is the same for all children. So, for instance, no child can sit up before acquiring head control.
4. As a rule a baby has to lose a primitive reflex movement before he can acquire a skill. In other words he must lose the grasp reflex before he can voluntarily grasp an object. Similarly he must lose the kick reflex before he can walk.
5. Progress to a specific activity is quite often made from generalized activity. For instance, walking is really a refinement of the purposeless leg movements of the six-month-old baby.
6. There is no doubt that a child's personality affects the age at which he reaches his milestones. Independent, determined children practice new activities more than others and master them earlier. Outgoing, gregarious children often have a strong desire to communicate and develop speech earlier than others.

The age at which a child acquires skills is decided not only by his own character aptitudes, but depends also on the behavior of others and on his environment. Like ourselves, a baby acquires a skill more easily if given the chance to practice and encouraged to do so, especially if all his efforts are applauded. Lack of opportunity and encouragement account in large part for the retarded physical, intellectual and social development of some children brought up in institutions. It may show as early as three months and be responsible for lateness in speaking.

Having said that, generalization on children's progress is not without its dangers, and having accepted that there are variations from the average which, though very wide, are not abnormal, it is possible to draw up rough guidelines as to how and when children reach the stages or 'milestones' of development. But don't expect all or even more than one skill to proceed simultaneously. And it's worth remembering that when a new skill is being acquired other previously learned ones tend to regress. So speech can slow down when a child is learning to balance on two legs. Lulls and spurts are common and normal. In a spurt a child may make up for a slow start and pass his peers. In a lull a child's body continues to mature and when he returns to the lost skill he may make astonishing progress very quickly.

Masturbation

Part of a child's natural physical development includes increasing awareness of his or her sex organs and the pleasure that comes with manipulating them. At about five or six months, when a baby is learning to hold things, it's quite natural for a boy to grasp at such an accessible part of his own body as his penis. However, at this age, it's very rare for children to fondle themselves purposefully. A little later they may bring themselves pleasure by rubbing their thighs together or rocking back and forwards or rubbing themselves against something. True masturbation may start in either sex from about the age of four or when, for instance, a boy realizes that an erection may be pleasurable. At about this time he may draw your attention to his erect penis, saying that it's big or sore; you can respond quite coolly by telling him that it will go down soon. If he retracts the foreskin you are only pointing out the truth if you say that it might be sore afterwards. Four and five year olds commonly exhibit curiosity in the genital parts of other boys and girls and, as part of this, naturally examine and compare with each other.

In very nearly all children these activities are absolutely normal and nothing fearful will happen as a result of them. Far more harm is done by rigid parental attitudes. It is quite wrong to scold children for masturbation, to make them feel ashamed if caught (they will only continue to masturbate in secret) or to fuss over it (they will soon learn to use it as an attention-seeking device). They should be distracted or ignored. Rarely, masturbation is associated with an infection of the skin around the penis or vagina or of the urine, and this should be treated by your doctor. In a boy it's usually because he's proud of his penis, or he needs pleasure after a frightening experience, or he needs reassurance about his own penis after noticing he's different from girls. Children may masturbate out of boredom, or because they are unhappy and need to console themselves, or just because it feels nice.

Learning to Speak and Communicate

0–6 months	Even at four or six weeks your baby will watch you when you speak to him and may open and close his mouth as though attempting to make a responsive sound. Around eight weeks he greets overt friendly overtures with smiles. By twelve weeks most babies register pleasure with squeals and gurgles. At sixteen weeks he laughs when pleased. As six months approaches he may blow bubbles and push out his tongue in imitation of speech. May try to imitate a simple vowel sound like *oo, ee.*
7–8 months	Occasionally but by no means meaningfully, he comes out with simple syllables like *ga, da, ba.* Will try to attract your attention playfully by making a noise like coughing.
9–12 months	May try to combine syllables like *ba-ba.* By a year he is normally saying his first word with meaning and this is largely a question of repetition. Will say first the word he hears most often, frequently *da-da* or an attempt at *hello.*
15–18 months	Is starting to say more and more words with meaning. If he wants something he will stand near it and shout for your attention and point. May bob his head by way of saying thank you. Will burble away to himself with sounds that mimic conversation but are his personal nonsense language.
2 years	By now he may be trying to join words together into phrases. May repeat words said to him. Can make very simple requests. Distinguishes in speech between himself *I* and others *you.* Is becoming a chatterer.

NB: All dates are approximate.

Learning and Understanding

Newborn   Your newborn baby likes warmth and gentleness and dislikes bright lights and loud noises. His eyes may move at your voice or attempt to follow your face.

4 weeks   Will watch you and even open and close his mouth when you talk to him, stop crying when you pick him up.

6 weeks   First responsive smiles are seen, and his eyes will begin to follow you or a moving toy.

8 weeks   It takes a few seconds for him to see something held above him, but then his eyes will follow it from side to side.

3 months   By this time he notices a toy immediately. Smiles when you speak and sometimes squeals with pleasure. Curiosity and interest become obvious.

4 months   Becomes excited when he sees the breast or bottle or toys. Laughs and chuckles. Likes to be propped up and turns his head at a sound.

6 months   Begins to take an interest in his mirror image. If he drops something he looks and reaches for it. Food preferences begin to show.

8 months   Is beginning to know his name and understand *No*. May cough to attract your attention. Reaches for things he wants.

9 months   May try to stop you washing his face. Starts to concentrate on toys and games. Will handle toys carefully and turn them over and over.

10 months   Is able to learn to clasp his hands, and possibly wave bye bye. Is beginning to show understanding of a few words and simple statements.

11 months   Likes playing peekaboo. Loves dropping things to have them picked up. Loves to shake things that rattle. Likes making noises with pots and pans for instance.

1 year   Will repeat anything that makes you laugh and enjoys looking at simple books with you. May hold up his arms as you undress him. Understands familiar words like *drink, bath, ball*. May even say two or three words with meaning.

15 months May show he wants to feed himself, brush his hair. Will kiss on request and will enjoy new skills like drinking from a cup. Will try to imitate your daily tasks like dusting and understands quite complex sentences.

18 months Will point to pictures of dogs and ducks, and can recognize and say *duck*. Knows parts of the body, like *foot* and *nose* and *Mummy's nose*. Will bring things if asked.

21 months Will take you to show you things. Likes scribbling with a pencil. Understands and obeys a variety of requests.

2 years Will play quite creatively on his own. May try to make up and down strokes with a pencil. Is learning the names of familiar objects and toys.

2¼ years Will try to build cars or trains with bricks. Tries to repeat new words when encouraged. Can say his first name. Is becoming increasingly negative. Uses the word *No* more often; disagrees with you, defies you.

2½ years Will draw horizontal and vertical lines and can name some common objects. Loves helping and will put things away for you. Can repeat his full name. Is noticing his sex organs.

2¾ years Tries unsuccessfully to draw a circle. Is beginning to ask questions. Knows what sex he is. Is beginning to learn rhymes and understands numbers.

3 years Will join other children playing. Knows one or two rhymes. Can almost draw a circle. Is beginning to count. Can distinguish such words as *on, under, behind*.

NB: All dates are approximate.

Learning to Control the Head

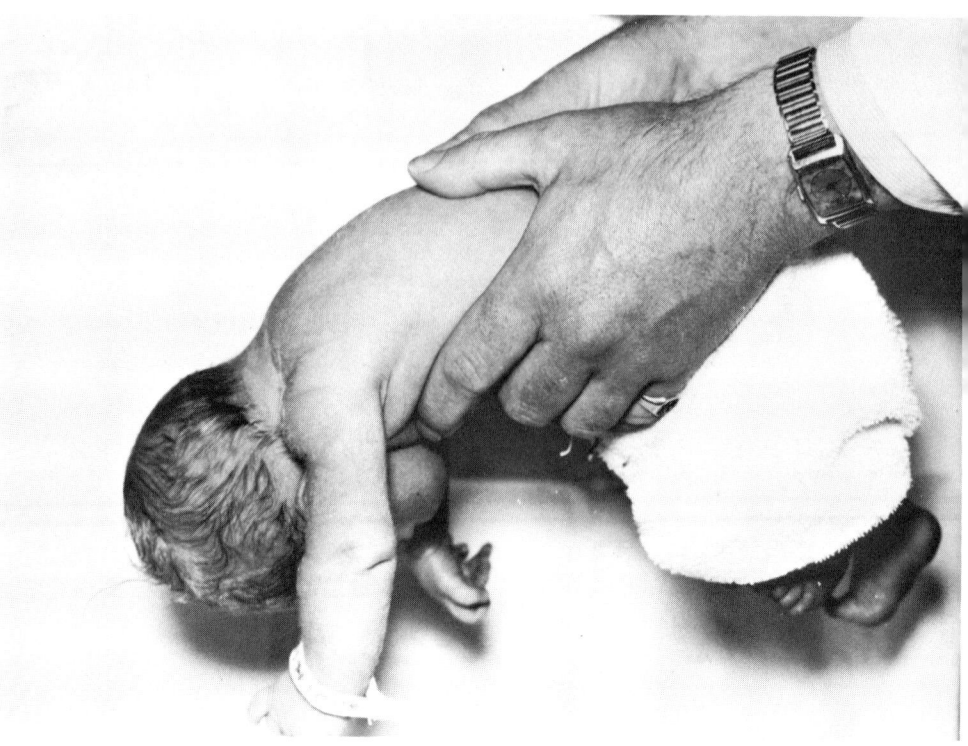

Newborn When held horizontal the head drops, and when lifted the head lags behind the rest of the body.

Eight weeks The neck muscles are getting stronger and he can hold his head slightly above the plane of his body.

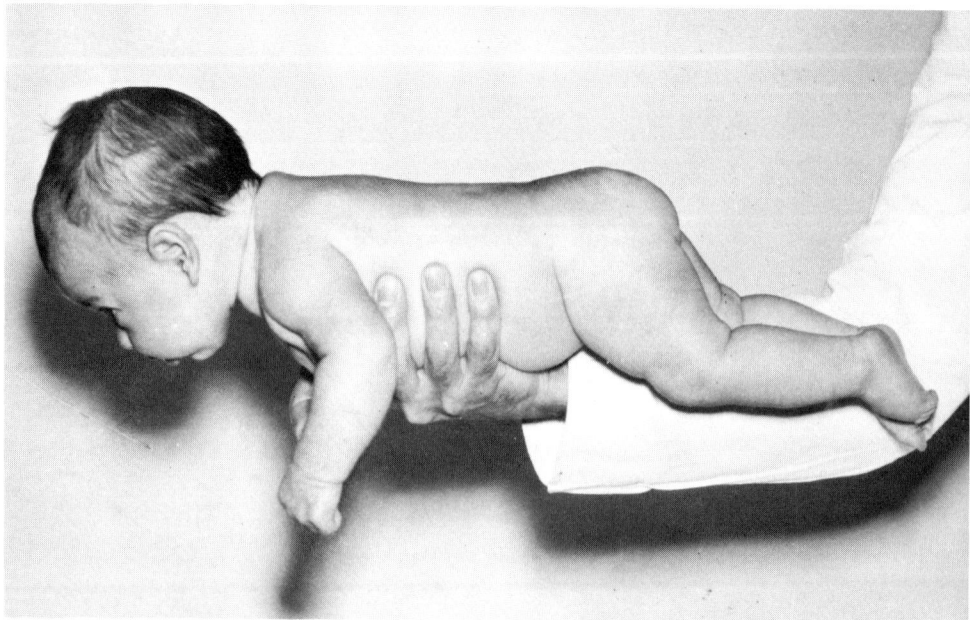

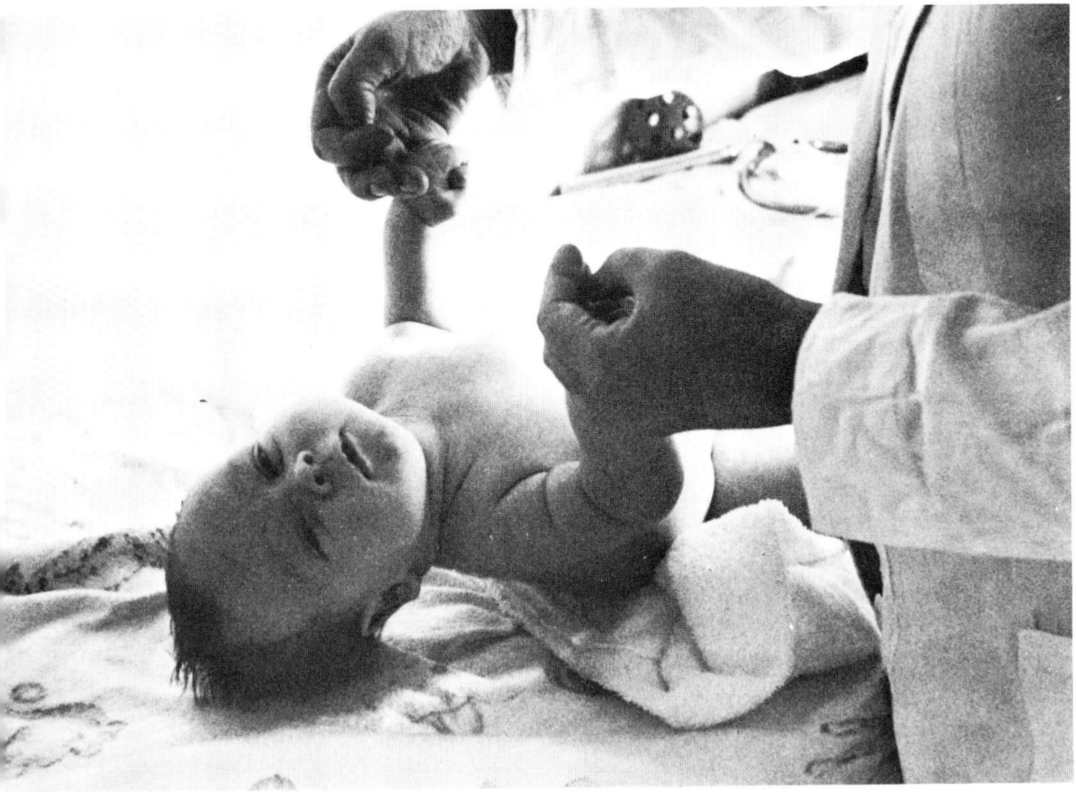

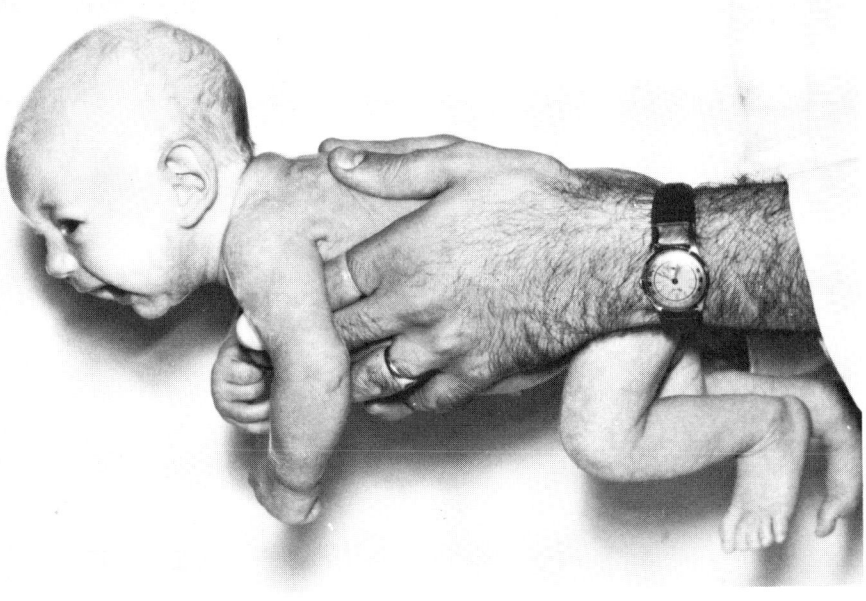

Six weeks When lifted from a lying position the baby can just hold his head in line with his body.

Twelve weeks The neck muscles are strong enough and the baby's coordination good enough to allow the head to be held quite high.

Learning to Sit Up

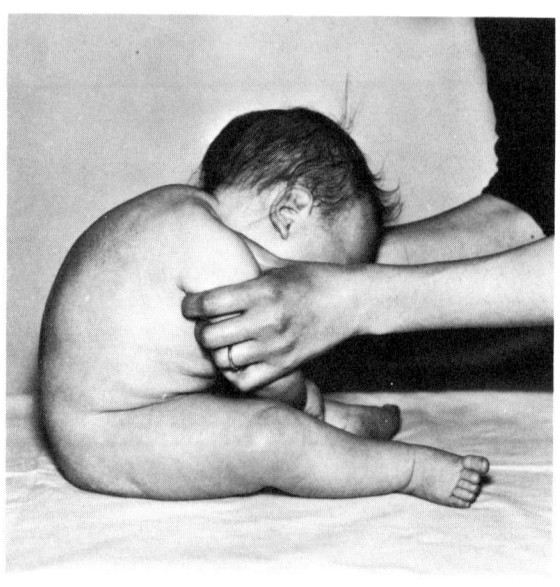

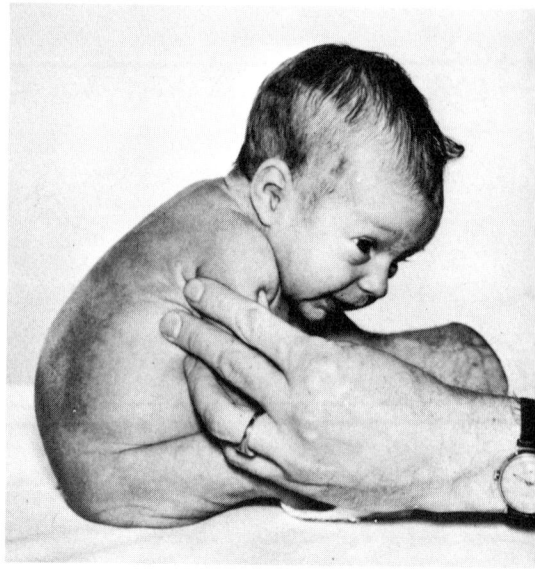

Newborn Your baby cannot sit at all without support, is wobbly and collapses in a few seconds; and the body keeps its curled-up shape.

One month The baby is a little steadier and might ho up the head for a moment, but the back is still rounded.

Seven months By this time he will be starting to sit on his own through supporting himself with his hands, often with them placed forward on the floor.

Eight months Your baby will almost certainly be sitting occasionally, quite straight and without support.

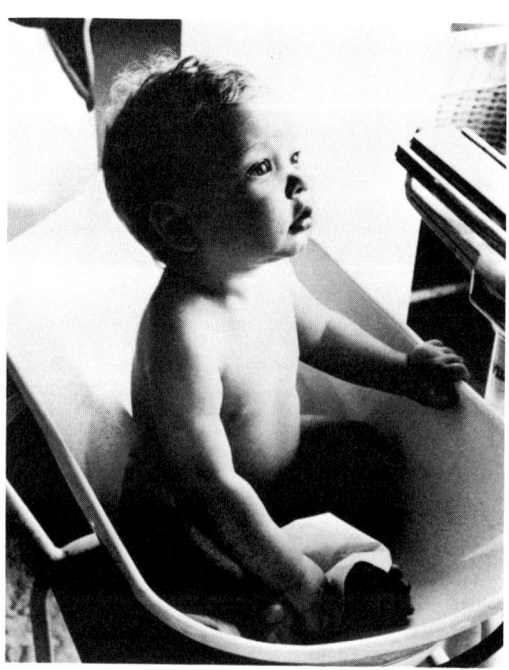

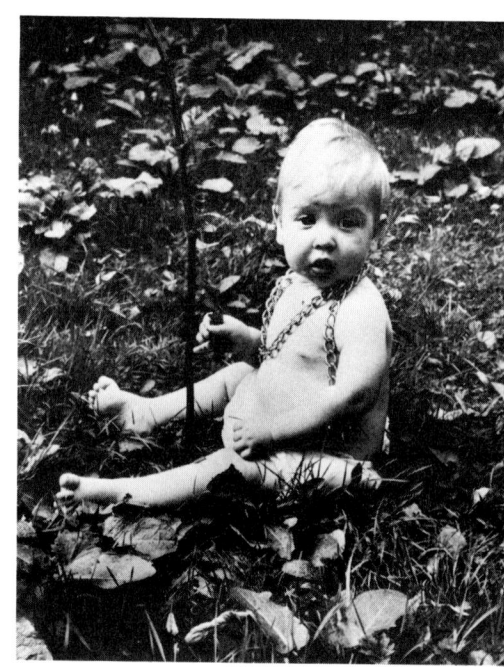

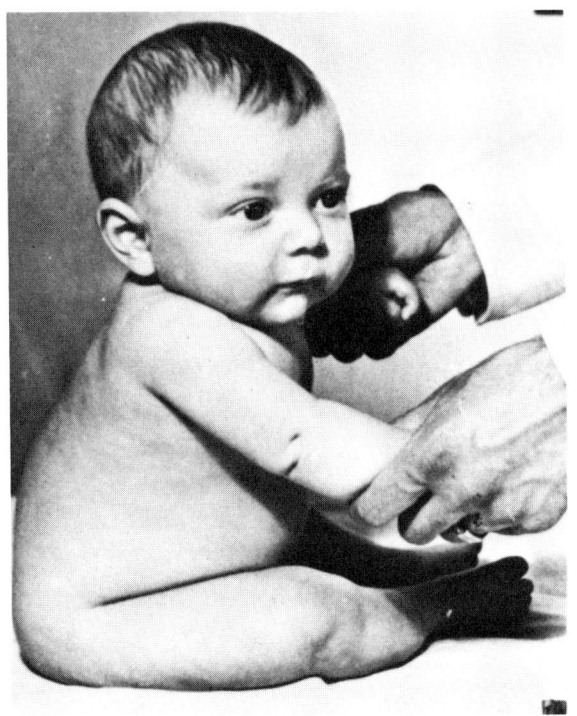

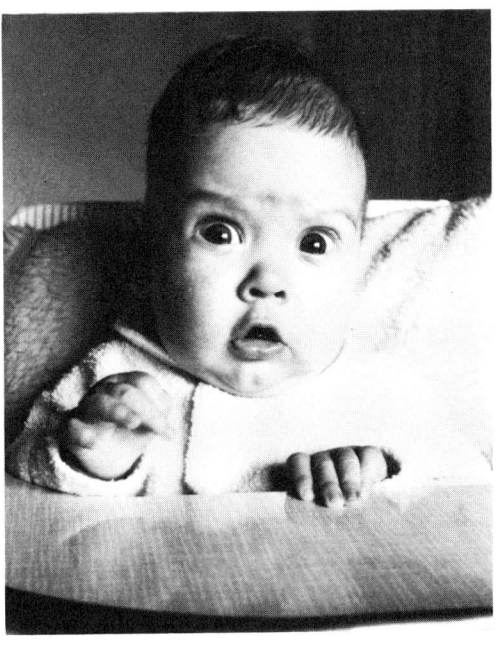

Four months Will probably manage to sit with the head held up if you support the arms. The upper part of the back will be almost straight but the lower part is still rounded.

Six months With cushions as a prop your baby may enjoy sitting up in a high chair.

Nine months May even be courageous enough to reach out to a - toy, or animal friend, from a sitting position.

Ten to twelve months Is starting to swing around from the waist so that she can see about her.

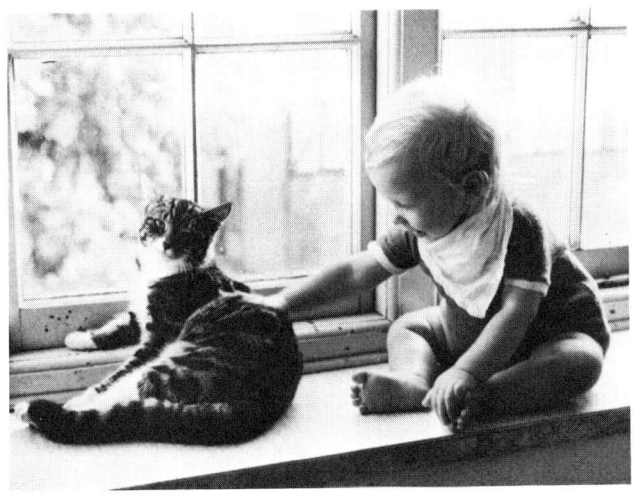

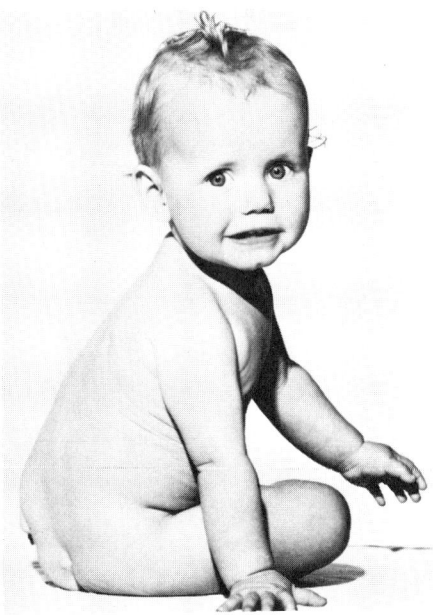

Learning to Crawl

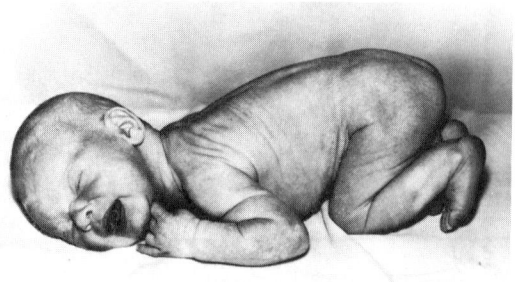

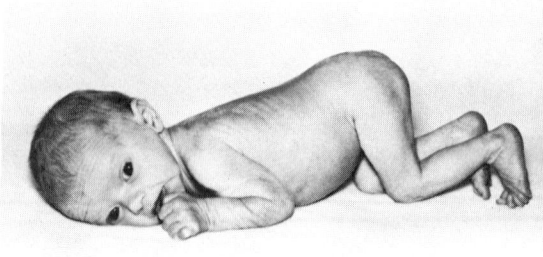

Newborn Your new baby lies with bottom in the air, legs drawn up under the body and the head on one side.

One month Now the chin is barely off the bed and one leg is starting to stretch out behind.

Six months Bends her knees up with a jerk and straightens them again. Reaches forward with her hands and can support her weight on her arms.

Seven to eight months Will try to take her weight on only one outstretched arm.

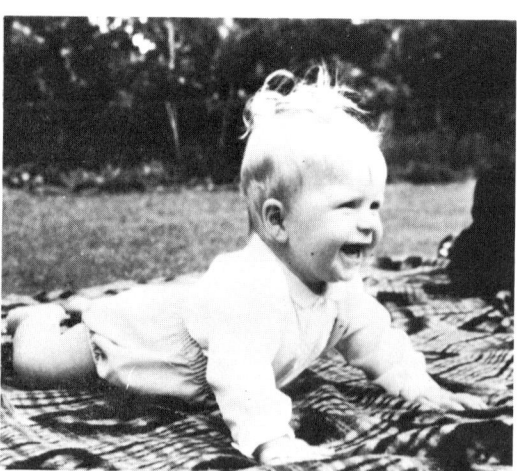

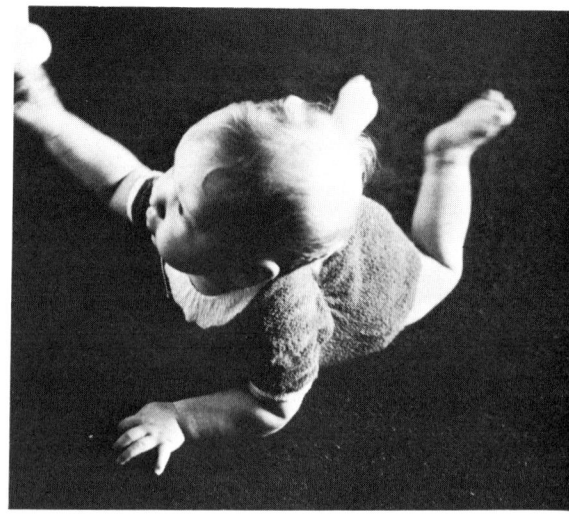

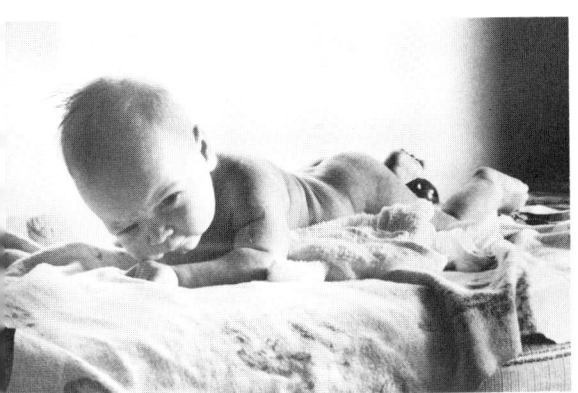

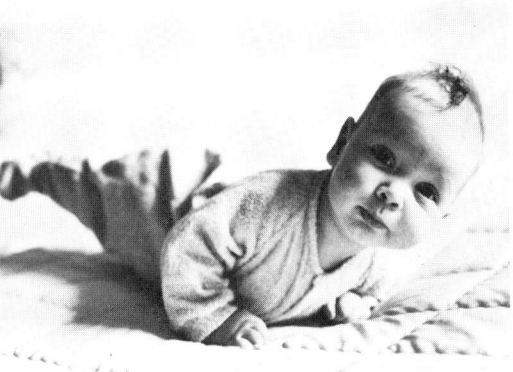

Two months Can by now straighten out both legs. Head is held up at an angle from the body.

Four months Will kick his legs up and down and try to hold his chest off the bed.

Nine to ten months Will try to pull himself forward with his tummy still on the floor.

Eleven to twelve months Your baby can get the tummy off the floor and creep. By a year old he or she may be on all fours.

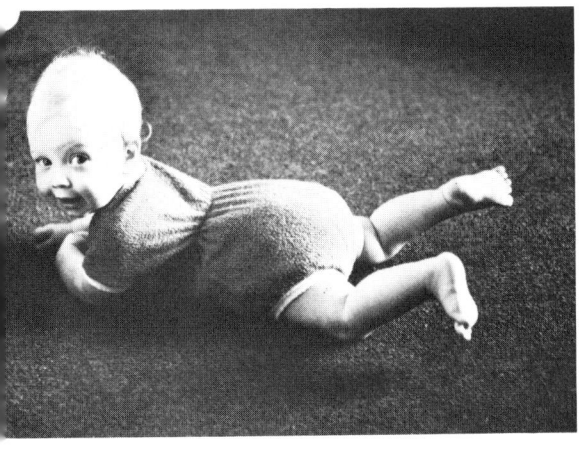

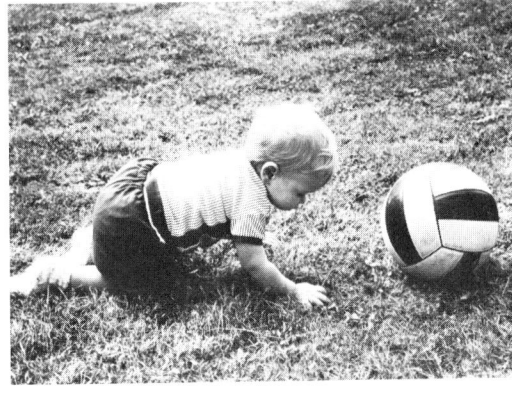

Learning to Walk

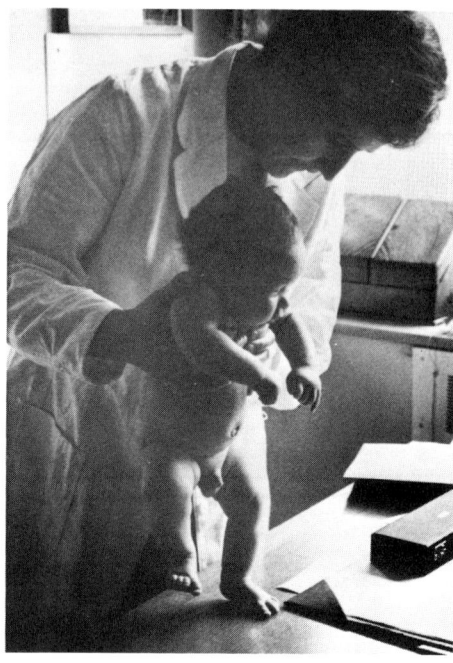

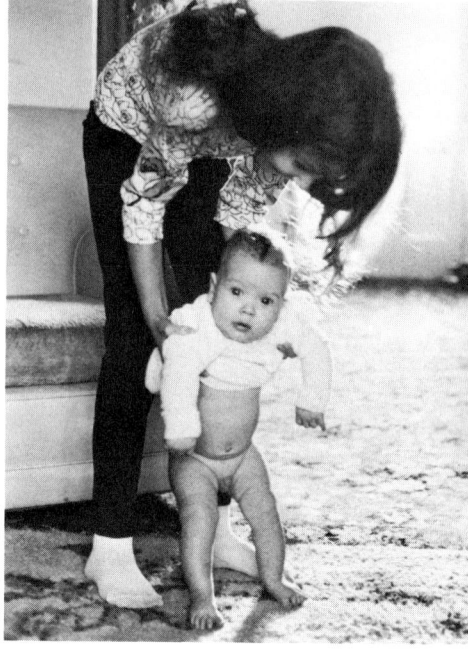

Three months Will momentarily take his weight if you hold him and let his feet touch the ground.

Six months If you help him to balance he will take most of his weight, though the knees are still bent.

Eleven to thirteen months Holding first both your hands then only one, she will probably try her first few steps and may stand on her toes if supported.

Thirteen to fifteen months May momentarily stand by himself, reach out to a support, then take a step.

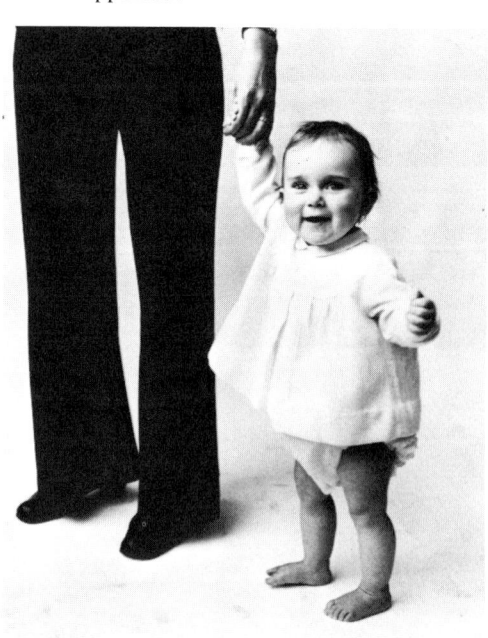

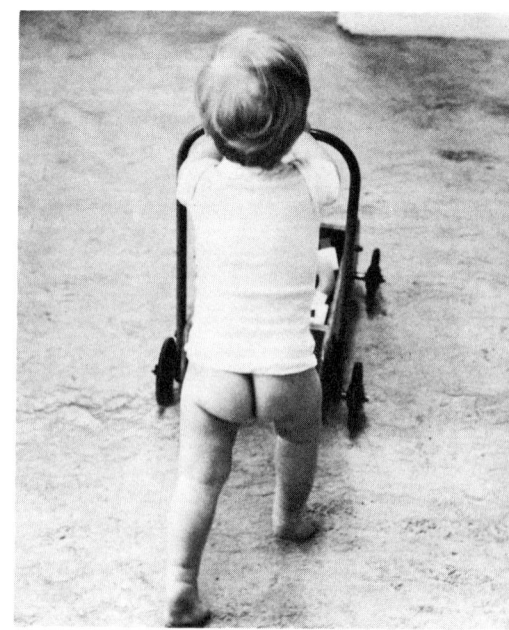

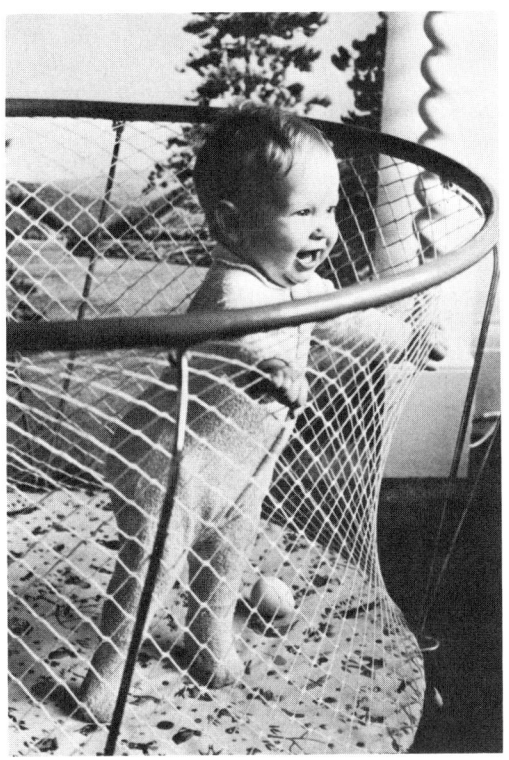

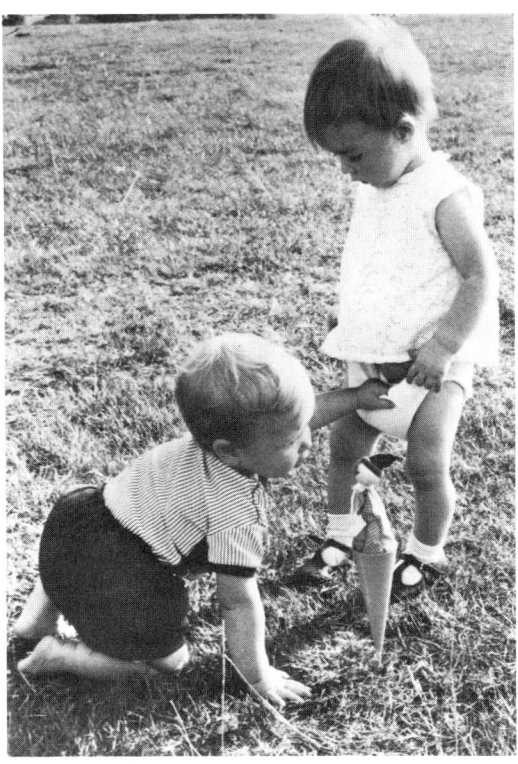

Nine months About now she may try standing while holding on to the furniture.

Ten to eleven months They will be trying to pull themselves up to a standing position.

Fifteen to eighteen months Will begin to walk without support, elbows held up, feet wide apart.

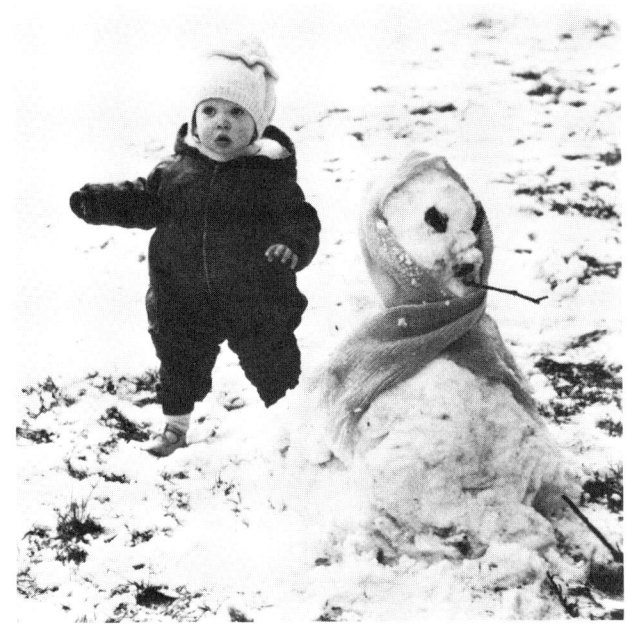

Learning to Walk (CONTINUED)

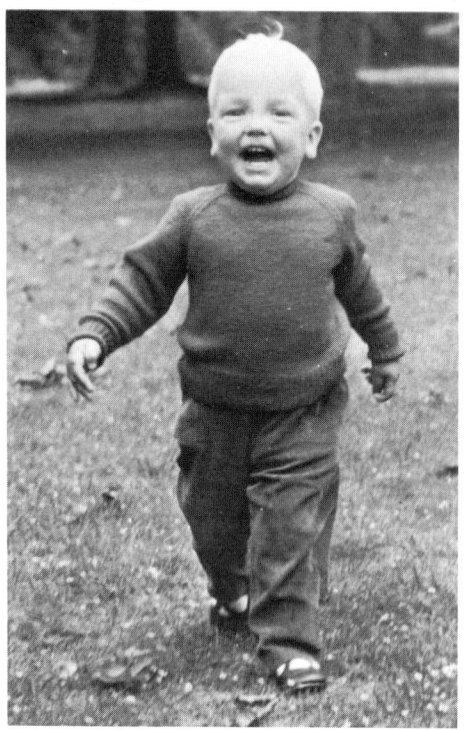

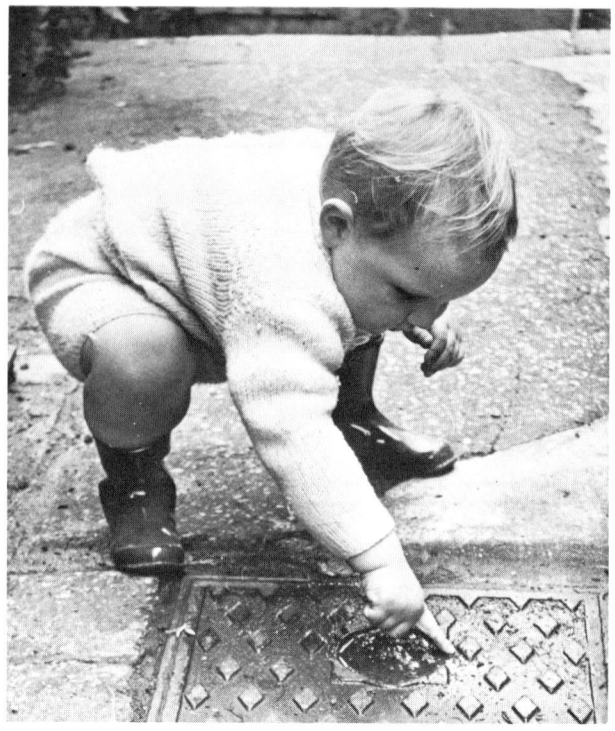

Eighteen to twenty months Their walking becomes steadier, arms now by their sides. They may attempt to walk upstairs.

Twenty-one to twenty-four months Will probably be able to bend down and pick things up without falling over.

Three years Their balance is so good that they can stand momentarily on one foot.

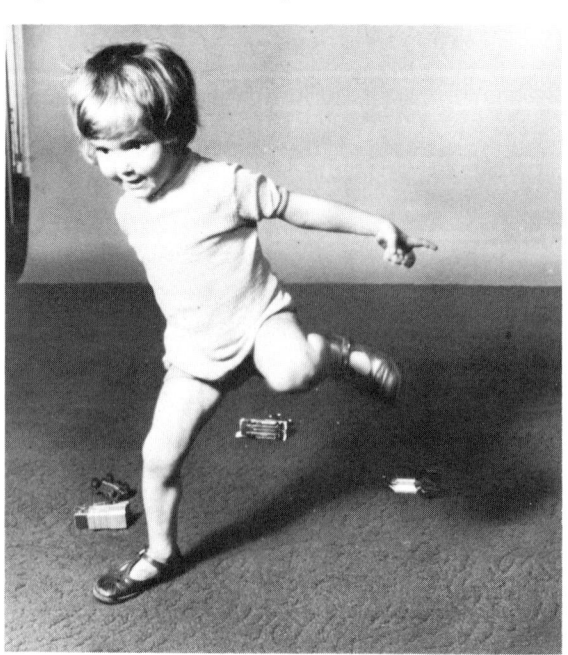

Learning to Use the Hands

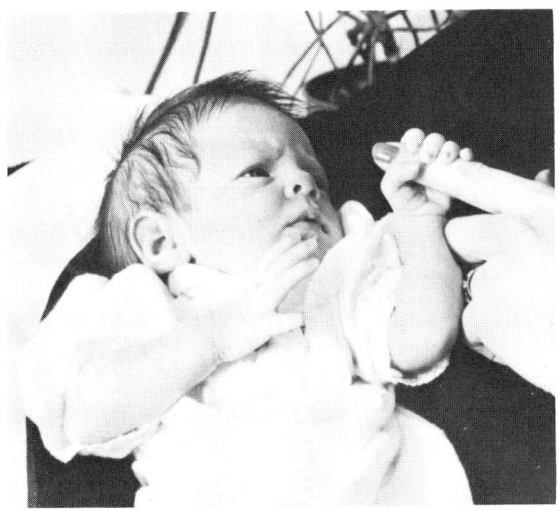

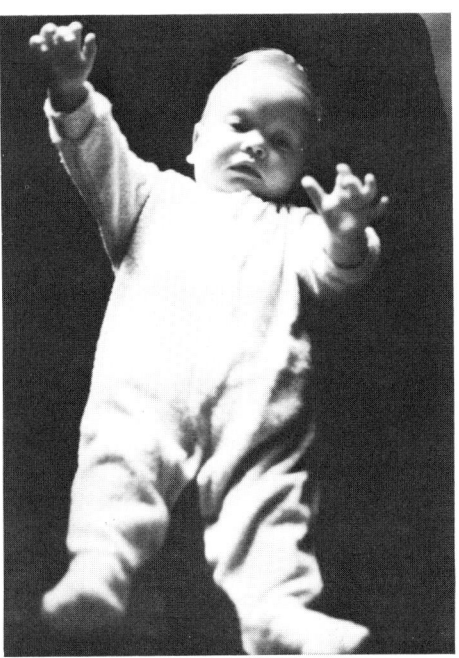

ewborn Your new baby has quite a strong grip and will old your finger tightly. This is the grasp reflex.

Three to four months The hands are now open most of the time. She studies them and examines the movements of her fingers. Reaches for things but misses them and will shake a rattle if it is put in her hands.

Five to six months Will grasp most things with the whole hand, holding them in the palm. Babies love feeling things and will crumple paper, splash water and may even hold a bottle. When lying on their backs they may grasp their toes. They will drop one cube if offered a second.

Eight to nine months May try to pass a toy from one hand to the other. Will start to put everything in his mouth and may try to feed himself with a rusk or piece of apple. Is probably banging things on the table.

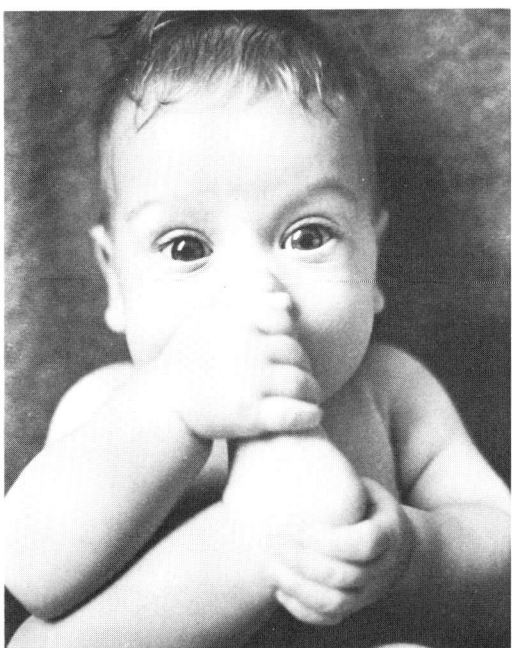

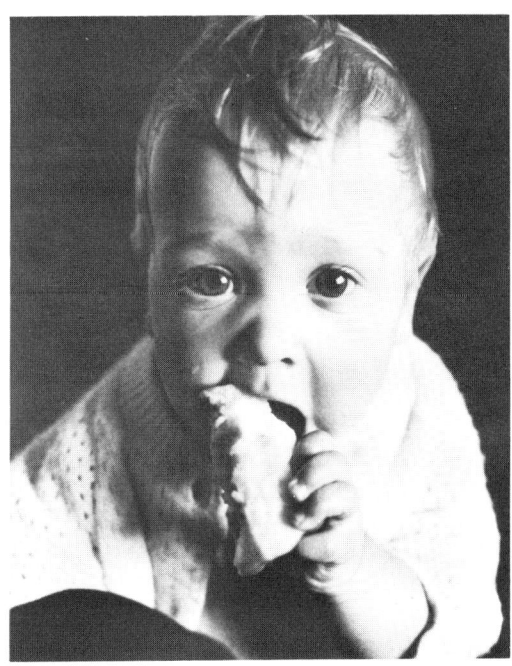

Learning to Use the Hands (CONTINUED)

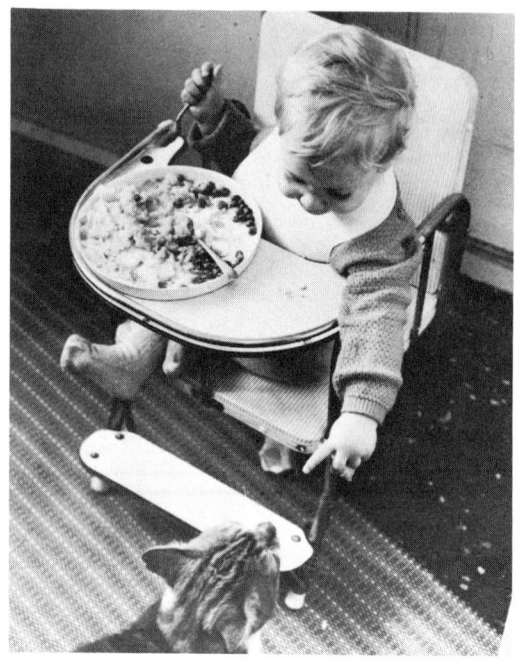

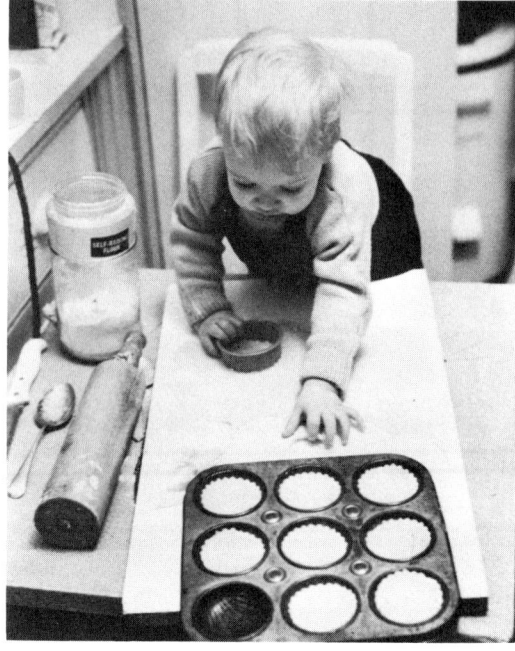

Ten to eleven months When babies reach for something they will lead with the index finger, as though pointing at it. They start to drop things purposely. They may be able to pick up something small, say a pea, with the finger and thumb.

One year Will be mastering the adult grip — between finger and thumb. Will give you something if you ask for it and may even roll a ball across the floor to you.

Eighteen months Is starting to build a tower of bricks, manipulate his food with a spoon and turn over the pages of a book two or three at a time. May try to open and close a zipper if shown how.

Two years They can just about turn a door handle or unscrew a loose lid, and they try very hard to put on their shoes and socks. They love washing and drying their hands.

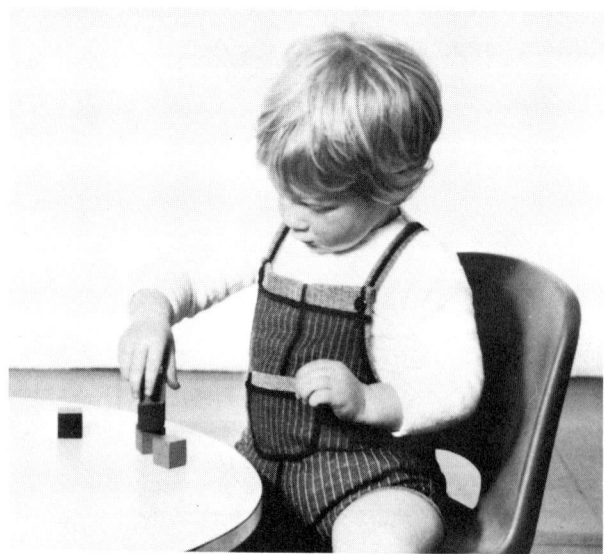

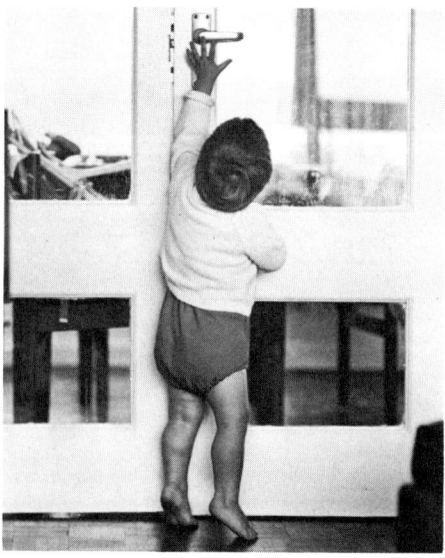

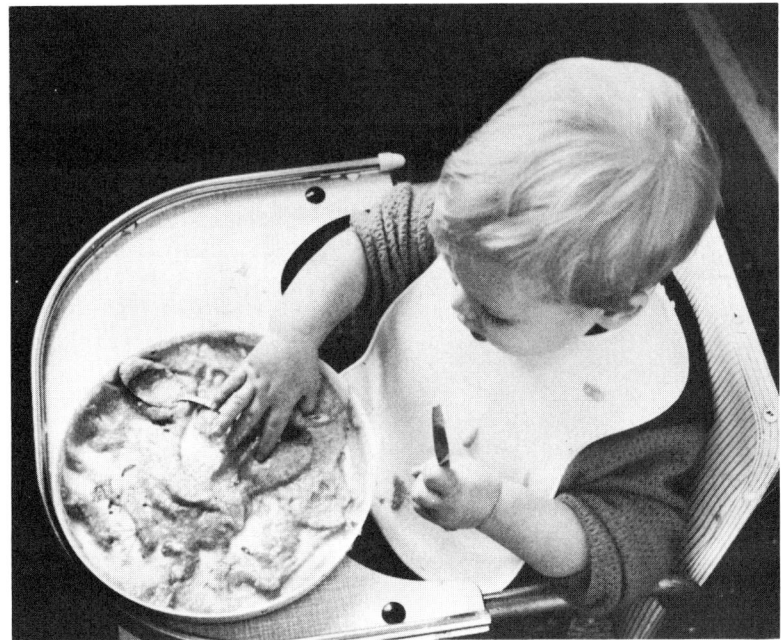

Thirteen to fifteen months May be able to hold two small objects in one hand, trying to make marks with a pencil, and putting one brick on top of another. May be starting to take off his shoes.

Three years They can build a tower of up to nine bricks, try to dress and undress themselves, and can sometimes manage to undo front buttons. They can carry a plate to and from the table and love helping with household chores and concentrating on games.

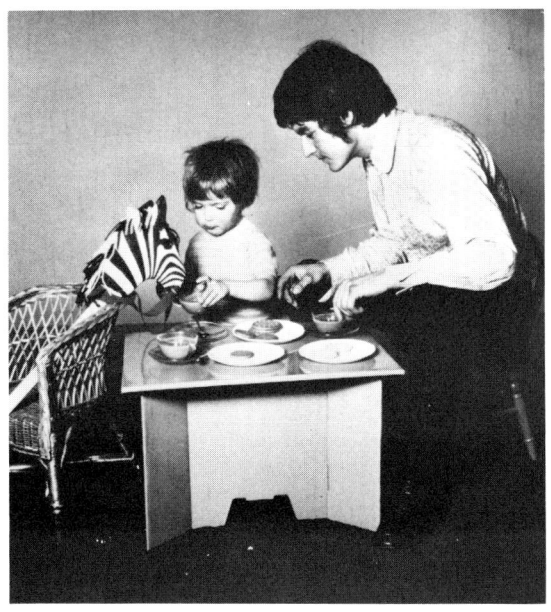

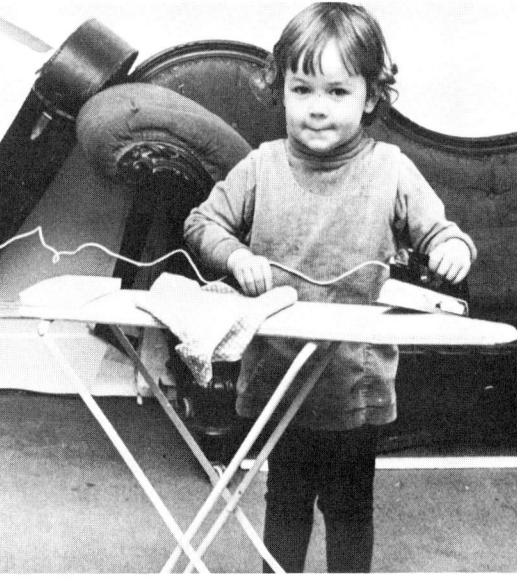

Appearance of First Teeth

The appearance of teeth is so variable (occasionally babies are born with a tooth and yet it's quite normal to have none at a year) that to put times on their eruption can be misleading. They do, however, usually erupt in the order shown below.

1. Lower front tooth (teeth)
2. Upper front tooth (teeth)
3. Upper side tooth
4. Lower side tooth
5. Upper first molar
6. Lower first molar
7. Upper eye teeth
8. Lower eye teeth
9. Lower second molars
10. Upper second molars

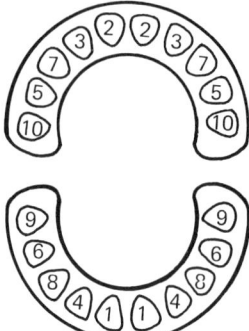

8 Bowel and Bladder Control

In the words of one of the most eminent British pediatricians, Prof. R. S. Illingworth, "toilet training" should always be "placid painless potting." This means that parents should remain placid at all costs and avoid causing any sort of pain (emotional as well as physical) to the child. Inflexible routines are out. It is quite wrong to expect children to conform to your ideas of bowel regularity — they may not be physiologically equipped to do so. It is quite wrong to force children to stay on their potties until they've performed to your satisfaction. This will only alienate them from parents as well as the potties. It's quite wrong to entice them to stay on their potties with bribes, games, and your company, as they will fast learn that they have been given an infallible attention-seeking device. It's quite wrong to threaten, punish, shame or ridicule your child, as it will encourage him to use your concern as a weapon against you. It's quite wrong to give a child an enema or a suppository to induce a bowel movement — plenty of roughage (brown bread, fruit, green vegetables) in the diet or a mild aperient like milk of magnesia will keep the motions soft and as regular as they should be. It is quite wrong to expect too much too soon and then scold the child for accidents; that is plain unfair. It is quite wrong to try to *train* a child.

Somewhere or other the word 'train' crept into child-care language, and as far as sphincter control is concerned it is very dangerous. You cannot *train* children, you can only help them when they are developmentally ready. And when a child is developmentally ready varies enormously from child to child. The first step to getting it right is to gauge when a child becomes able to control bowels and bladder voluntarily, and how the body and mind mature sufficiently to implement control. Bladder control is a very complex physiological mechanism that involves not just the muscles and nerves of the bladder and bowel, but the brain as well. The inherent instinct of a full bladder is to empty itself. As we learn not to void urine sponta-neously, the brain countermands this reflex and we wait. When, at a convenient moment, we decide we want to empty the bladder, the brain has to cancel the first order to hold on, and gives the signal to let go. So it's a three-step intellectual process. What actually hap-pens in the bladder is no less complicated.

How the Bladder Works

The bladder is made up of a bag of muscle whose outlet is controlled by a tight band of muscle fibers called a sphincter, running round the neck of the bag. The muscular action of the bag and the sphincter is controlled by two sets of nerves, the sympathetic and the parasym-pathetic fibers. It is the job of the sympathetic nerves to stop leaks, so when they stimulate the bladder the muscular bag relaxes to al-low filling and the sphincter contracts to prevent urine escaping. The parasympathetic does the opposite — it empties the bladder. Stimu-lation of parasympathetic nerves brings about contraction of the bladder walls and relaxation, causing opening of the sphincter and expulsion of urine.

Now when you consider that some eighteen-month-old babies, whose nervous systems are only just mature enough to carry mes-sages to and from the brain, are being asked to master this compli-cated mechanism, it's not surprising that they find it a difficult and sometimes impossible request. They simply do not possess the equipment until they are developmentally ready and it's quite unjust to make demands prematurely.

When Is a Child Developmentally Ready?

Many babies do in fact empty their bowel and bladder during or soon after a meal as early as two or three months. Some mothers delightedly assume they're on the road to clean diapers and dry nights. This is not so. Small babies and their mothers are simply the beneficiaries of the babies' reflexes. In other words the baby has no control over the bladder or bowel at all. Voluntary control rarely begins before fifteen to eighteen months and often later, girls normally earlier than boys. Your baby will tell you very clearly that voluntary control is beginning and you should wait for him or her to give you the sign.

The first indication babies give is that they notice when they pass urine; they may stop and point to their diaper or attract your attention with a sound or shout. They hardly ever do this before fifteen months, and may not until they are over two. As they get older and their awareness increases, they will tell you no, they don't want to pass urine, if you ask. The next stage is when they alert you to the fact that they are going to urinate, but only seconds before and they cannot wait. As they grow older they master this urgency to pass urine and gradually allow you sufficient time to take down their clothes and place them on the potty. This happens by no means every time at first and there will undoubtedly be accidents that should be ignored or made little of. By about two-and-a-half years babies will allow themselves time to go to the bathroom and pull their own clothes down. They may even try to reach the toilet themselves, especially if you make it easy for them by putting a very sturdy step in front of the toilet. Very soon they may show self-reliance by wishing to do everything for themselves and demand privacy that should be respected. So in a relatively few months they have passed through the stages of just noticing the passage of urine, then the desire to pass urine, then, as their fastidiousness increases, the ability to wait for quite a long time.

Bowel control normally comes before bladder control. A study has shown that by two-and-a-half years approximately 90 percent of girls and 75 percent of boys have complete bowel control, even to the extent of going to the bathroom alone. The same study showed more than half the children at that age were still wet at night, though they could go without a diaper during the day. Bladder control at night comes last of all. A two-and-a-half-year-old child cannot hold urine for much longer than four to five hours, and often less. By the age of three, encouraging your child to pass urine just before you go to bed will help him to be dry in the morning. This should never be done if it distresses your child and accidents must be forgiven light-heartedly. Many children, boys especially, still occasionally wet the bed at well over the age of four. A change of surroundings or routine, an illness or unhappiness may cause bed-wetting to recur. So what should you do? If you remember that helpfulness and sympathy are the key words and try to get rid of the idea that you are training your child, it's mainly common sense. You can help by dressing your child in convenient clothes that can be taken down easily and quickly, so that accidents due to urgency can be avoided. As soon as your child is older you can build self-reliance by showing him how to take down his own clothes, how to use the toilet, and how to step up to it if it's high. A child will probably become very proud of these new skills and take pride in staying clean and dry.

Don't try to take diapers off too soon. The time to attempt this is after your child has learned to show you clearly that he wants to pass urine and can wait a few moments for you to get him to the potty or toilet. Training pants to my mind have no place in this routine. First, they suggest a training program, which I am against. Second, if he's dry he doesn't need them, and if he still can't wait he should be in a diaper. So the first step is waiting for him to do without a diaper while he's awake during the day.

Next, you can try taking off the diaper during your child's daytime nap, encouraging him to empty the bladder before you put him down. If he manages to stay dry, do praise him. If he doesn't, never, never scold him. Don't rush to take off his nighttime diaper until he can stay dry after being toileted last thing at night. It's a mistake to think you are 'training' your child to empty his bladder at ten or eleven o'clock — most children don't even wake when you're doing this. In fact it's a mistake to wake them. They often have difficulty getting back to sleep and are tired the next day. Quite often they're upset and cry. This only teaches them that going to the toilet is associated with feeling unhappy. It is very unlikely that a child will be able to remain dry from midnight to morning before two and a half, and three is a more realistic age to bear in mind. If it does come earlier than that, think of it as a bonus.

Once your child can stay dry during the night, try taking off the diaper and help him by putting a potty next to the bed. Encourage him to manage on his own. It's important that you help your child at this stage. It's quite a big step for him to stop relying on you and take the responsibility for himself. Accidents will of course still occur, so minimize your work and his anxiety by keeping a small rubber sheet on top of the ordinary sheet, and then put an additional sheet over that. This top sheet can be whipped off and washed if it gets wet. Make sure that nightwear is free of buttons and zippers so that the child can pull trousers down without trouble during the night. And never forget the golden rule — avoid a confrontation with your child. Force will accomplish nothing, gentleness and understanding invariably pays off.

Occasionally a child's progress to sphincter control is seriously interrupted or, having achieved control, the child regresses to an earlier stage. This is nearly always a sign of emotional disturbance or there is a psychological cause such as rejection. The exacerbating factor may be obvious, like the advent of a new baby when the older child feels rejected and engages in all sorts of attention-seeking behavior, including wetting and soiling clothes. Starting nursery school, moving to a new house, or the absence of parents could all stimulate the same pattern of behavior. If none of these things has happened, the possibility of infection should be eliminated by your doctor and your child examined if necessary.

There is no doubt that some perfectly normal children acquire bladder control later than others and present difficult problems to their parents. Often there is a history in the family of lateness in acquiring sphincter control. Most doctors believe, however, that there is no need to contemplate full investigation of this difficulty before a child is three years old if wet during the day, and five years old if still wet at night, though your general practitioner may ask you to take along a specimen of urine so that he can look at it. Medicines rarely help in this situation unless an infection is present, and assiduous efforts on the part of the parents probably only serve to aggravate. The best you can do is to be especially kind and helpful and take things slowly.

If a child's diet is rich in roughage, true constipation, i.e. a lazy bowel, rarely occurs. Constipation in a child is nearly always triggered off by the child who for one reason or another holds back a stool. In a desire to do this the child ignores the call to stool and as a result the rectum becomes insensitive to distension. It and the lower bowel may dilate and become loaded with hard feces. This in turn may irritate the lining of the bowel, which responds by producing mucus, and this may appear as watery diarrhea. So the paradox of constipation with diarrhea appears. Obviously it's best to prevent constipation from developing, but if it does you will need expert advice from your doctor and possibly special treatment.

For your part you have to help your child to overcome this difficulty and encourage him to respond to the call to stool. This nearly always happens after a full meal, quite often after breakfast. You can help by leaving enough time between breakfast and setting off for school for going to the bathroom in a leisurely fashion. Bear in mind that not all children need to empty their bowels every day and no harm will come to them if they don't.

Prolonged bed-wetting or nocturnal enuresis can be equally difficult for you and your child. Even knowing that bed-wetting eventually stops, it's quite natural for you to want to get over it quickly. More often than not your child is just as eager as you to help, but cannot. So again it's best for everyone if you try to stay cool and calm and minimize the problem. Putting pressure on your frustrated child will only make it harder for him. While the cause of nocturnal enuresis may be emotional there may be other causes that are out of your child's control, like an unusually small bladder, or a family trait that's been inherited, or unavoidable stress. (For further discussion, see page 151).

You can see that those parents who claim that they have never had a dirty diaper since their baby was six months old have been the beneficiaries of good luck and primitive reflexes. Most children who seem to have acquired early bowel control regress and have to pass through the maturing process I have described.

9 Common Childhood Illnesses

It's very unlikely that your child will negotiate the minefield of growing up without ever being ill, or for that matter without taking any form of medicine. I recently met a friend who had astonished her new doctor with the information that her two-year-old son had never received antibiotics. "It must be years since I've seen a two-year-old baby who has never had any of those medicines," said the doctor. Whether it was due to having a sensible mother, or a very attentive general practitioner, or just plain luck, is difficult to decide, but it's unlikely that your baby will be as lucky as my friend's child. Most caring parents observe their babies carefully, and without noting specific signs and symptoms you will know when your baby is ill. Almost the first decision you have to make is whether to call the doctor.

When to Call the Doctor

LOSS OF APPETITE
If your child is normally a good regular eater, loss of appetite is something that you should note. It's one of the first warnings that all is not well, regardless of the sort of illness your child is suffering from. In small children it's often due to an infection and needs your doctor's immediate attention. In the first weeks of life infants cannot afford to go without their food for very long and infections can quickly become serious.

VOMITING
Some children vomit effortlessly when a piece of food gets stuck or when they cough, and it never seems to bother them at all. But if vomiting is unusual it is always a serious sign.

DIARRHEA

A small baby with loose watery stools should always be treated promptly because she can quickly become dehydrated. There are many explanations for diarrhea in an older child, but if she has a temperature, abdominal pain, and seems ill, you should contact your doctor.

DIFFICULTY IN BREATHING

Regardless of when your child shows that she's having difficulty with breathing, you should get in touch with your doctor, *whatever the hour of day or night.* You may notice that she's breathing fast or having to work hard at breathing, or that she wheezes and the lower part of the rib cage is drawn in with every breath.

VERY HIGH TEMPERATURE

Children get hot and have a high temperature for many reasons, not all of which are serious, but if your child has a temperature over 38°C (100°F) and is obviously ill, or 103°F whether showing signs of illness or not, you should call your doctor. It's worth remembering that babies may be very ill indeed with a temperature that is *lower* than normal.

EMERGENCIES

A serious accident, particularly if your child loses consciousness or accidentally drinks or eats a poisonous substance, always warrants calling your doctor. It may be that he will refer you to a hospital. Take your child there immediately if you cannot contact your doctor quickly. Keep all your medicines well out of reach of your children. Have a lock fitted to the cabinet if it doesn't come with lock and key, and keep it locked at all times. And keep the telephone number of your nearest Poison Control handy.

IF YOU ARE WORRIED

As a junior doctor I very quickly learned that those whom I must take seriously were parents who were worried about their children. They *know.* If you feel that your child is not quite right, regardless of whether or not there is anything you can put your finger on, your doctor won't mind if you seek reassurance.

112

Coughs, Colds and the Upper Respiratory System

In children the nose, sinuses, throat, ears, and upper chest are ana-
tomically closely related. Connections between various parts are
short, and they may be considered members of the one system. This
explains why a cold can often spread down on to the chest and
cause bronchitis, or a sore throat can progress to an ear infection. In
adults, diseases of these various systems tend to remain separate
from one another. With children it isn't unusual for a runny nose to
progress to acute tonsillitis in only a few hours.

COLDS

Contrary to popular belief, a cold is not caused by going outside
with wet hair, wearing too little clothing on a freezing cold day or
being soaked to the skin in a rainstorm. These are old wives' tales.
The common cold is caused by a virus. At the present time doctors
have no way of killing off viruses, which is why there is no cure for
the common cold. The virus enters the body through the nasal passages and throat, causing inflammation of the lining membranes and
the well-known symptoms of runny nose and sore throat. It takes
the body's own defenses about ten days to overcome this invasion.
What is possibly more important, particularly in children, is that the
virus can weaken the body and allow secondary bacteria to multiply. The clear nasal discharge then becomes yellow. The tonsils and
adenoids may swell up and become septic, and your child will develop swollen glands in the neck. The tonsils, the adenoids, and the
glands are part of the body's defenses against infection, and during
the battle they may become swollen.

A cold is frequently accompanied by a cough because the mucus dripping down the back of the nose irritates the throat and your
child will cough to get rid of it. The younger the baby, the more she
is upset by a cold. Blockage of the nose doesn't allow the child to
breathe while feeding. You can alleviate this difficulty by using nose
drops that clear the nasal passages for long enough to enable the
baby to feed comfortably. Nose drops should never be used frequently over long periods because they can damage the lining of the
nose.

If you or any member of the close family has a cold, there is
very little chance of keeping it away from the baby. Whoever tends
the baby regularly, however, should wear a mask (available from

good drugstores), and a visitor to the house who has a cold must keep out of the baby's room. As a rule there is no need to call the doctor about a child who has a cold unless she has a high temperature, complains of earache or sore throat, and seems ill. In due course the body will overcome a cold infection itself. As children are less susceptible to the discomfort of a cold than adults, there is no need to give them the proprietary cold cures that we turn to with the first sneeze. You should certainly not give your child a nightly aspirin tablet to help her sleep, as aspirins have serious side effects and must only be used when necessary.

COUGHS

Coughing is very often part of an upper respiratory tract infection. There are two types of cough — the *productive* cough, when your child is using the cough reflex to clear mucus coming up from the chest or down from the back of the nose; and the *unproductive* cough, which is dry and irritating, with no useful purpose. It is important to make the distinction because a productive cough must never be suppressed with cough medicine. On the other hand, an unproductive cough can distress a child, keep him awake at night and even cause vomiting if the bout of coughing is particularly prolonged. It's good to suppress the second kind of cough. Keep by you a bottle of cough suppressant linctus prescribed by your doctor, which can be safely given to children. Persistent coughing in a small baby can be upsetting for the baby and worrying for the parent. It is always worth consulting your doctor to see if there is any form of specific treatment that would help. A postnasal drip is one of the commonest causes of night coughing. The nasal secretions drip into the back of the throat and set off the cough reflex. You can avoid this by turning your child on to the side or front.

TONSILS AND ADENOIDS

The tonsils are the watchdogs of the throat. In other words they trap bacteria and viruses, localize throat infections and sound the alarm bell to the rest of the body when an infection is present so that the body can prepare its defenses. The adenoids are at the back of the nose and perform the same function; consequently tonsils and adenoids are often bracketed together. They are most important to us in the first decade of life, for it is then that we meet most infectious illnesses and when our defenses must be strongest.

As they perform such a useful function, you may rightly ask why they are removed. It used to be very fashionable to take out Ts and As. It no longer is. The indications for surgical removal are very clearly defined, and most otolaryngologists would only agree to do so if your child was suffering from recurrent attacks of severe tonsillitis associated with ear infections and deafness. Even so, the tonsils are rarely removed before the age of four. Surprisingly a child rarely complains of a sore throat and acute tonsillitis may only be discovered when your doctor carries out a throat examination as part of the routine check of a sick child. Acute tonsillitis can be particularly severe when a virulent form of the streptococcus bacterium is the infecting agent. Your child may have a high swinging temperature, refuse food, cough a great deal, be unable to sleep and need a good deal of attention. Only your doctor can tell if antibiotics are indicated, and you must consult him. The most frequent complication associated with recurrent tonsillitis is an infection of the middle ear (otitis media). Germs can quite easily make their way up the Eustachian tube that connects the throat with the middle ear. Frequent attacks of otitis media may cause deafness and, if not treated rigorously, can lead to permanent damage of the eardrum.

EARACHE

If your child complains of earache it doesn't necessarily mean that there is something wrong with his ears, for pain from the throat, the teeth and the sinuses can be referred to the ears. The upper respiratory tract in small children is a system of interconnected compartments and any infection of any part may lead to ear trouble. Persistent earache or deafness, or pus coming from the ear, should cause you concern and send you immediately to your doctor. Enlarged or infected tonsils or adenoids may be the root cause and if this is so they should be removed. A serious ear infection may cause a fever, loss of appetite and even vomiting and diarrhea, and can mislead parents who are unaware of the connection. Most doctors are not as easily misled and will almost certainly prescribe antibiotics, possibly along with nose drops to aid drainage of the infection. Ear drops do no good at all as it is impossible for them to penetrate the ear drum and reach the seat of infection.

BRONCHITIS

Healthy children commonly get bronchitis, an inflammation of the air passages inside the lung. Inflammation usually results in the secretion of large amounts of mucus. This narrows the size of the bronchial tubes and can cause wheezing. As the mucus is cleared from the lungs, it causes a productive cough. Wheezing that comes on with a chest infection should not necessarily therefore be labeled as asthmatic. A real attack of asthma comes on suddenly for little reason whether an infection is present or not. Many very young babies (between four and ten percent) wheeze with even a slight chest infection and usually grow out of this tendency by the time they are five years old. The main aim in treating children with bronchitis should be to encourage them to cough. Don't expect your child to spit up phlegm like an adult — he will almost certainly swallow it. This is not a bad thing, for the stomach is quite a safe place for infected phlegm, but it may cause vomiting. Antibiotics may be given for the wheezy bronchitis of childhood, and antispasmodics that open up narrowed bronchial tubes can bring substantial relief.

CROUP

The symptoms of croup are a rasping cough, often accompanied by difficulty with breathing, each intake of breath being accompanied by a squeaky croaking sound. Croup is commonest between the ages of two and four. Quite often the susceptibility to it runs in families and it tends to recur. It is caused by inflammation of the vocal cords, which swell and leave only a narrow passageway for air to enter the windpipe. The air being drawn through the obstructed larynx makes the typical 'croup' sound and may result in labored breathing. If you see that your child is having difficulty with breathing you should call the doctor whatever the time of day or night. While waiting for the doctor to arrive you can do the following things to help your child:

1. Stay with your child to give her reassurance.
2. Stay calm; any anxiety you show may make her afraid and her breathing worse.
3. Sit her up; breathing can be more difficult if she's lying down.
4. Prop her up with pillows so that she can rest.
5. If her bedroom is centrally heated, open the windows a few inches to cool the air a little.
6. Better still, humidify the air with a vaporizer or by keeping a kettle on the boil in the room (if you do this, don't leave the room).

116

As croup may recur your doctor will probably give you instructions on how to deal with a possible future attack.

Abdominal Pain

Our mothers and grandmothers will tell us that a baby with abdominal pain will cry and draw the legs up. Unfortunately most babies draw up their legs when they cry, so you must look around for other signs that tell you whether your baby is ill or perfectly well. As a general rule, if your baby stops crying when you hold and comfort her and continues to take food normally, there is very little wrong with her. On the other hand, a baby who is off her food, who is vomiting or has diarrhea and who cries persistently and momentarily goes pale while crying needs prompt medical attention.

The older child will tell you she has a pain in her stomach, although she may not necessarily mean it. She may be feeling generally unwell and her ill feeling seems to center in the abdomen. She may, as already described, have an ear infection or tonsillitis with swollen glands. The degree of pain that your child is suffering is not necessarily an accurate index of how seriously ill she is, but if the pain appears to be severe and she seems ill, call your doctor immediately regardless of the hour. Don't wait to see if the pain goes away when your child has any combination of abdominal pain, vomiting, diarrhea and fever.

Vomiting

Vomiting is not the same as spitting, which is the effortless bringing up of small quantities of milk after feeding; neither is it the bringing up of phlegm that has collected at the back of the throat. Vomiting is the forcible emptying of the stomach contents. Children vary in their tendency to vomit, and some do it often without harmful effect. If vomiting is a rare event in your child's life, you should always be on the lookout for other signs of illness. There is very rarely anything wrong with the child who continues to eat, but if your child vomits persistently, refuses food and has other signs of abdominal disease such as diarrhea, you should seek your doctor's advice.

Diarrhea

Diarrhea means frequent, loose stools when there are signs that the intestines are hurrying the food along. A change of diet when you go on vacation may be sufficient cause. More serious causes are food poisoning or gastroenteritis. Diarrhea is dangerous in small babies because the intestine is not given time to absorb valuable water from the stool and severe dehydration can ensue. It needs very prompt medical treatment. If your child remains well, is perfectly happy and eats normally, there is no need to be concerned about the odd loose stool, but again if he is off his food or is vomiting, or there is blood in the stool, he needs prompt attention. Proprietary medicines have little place in the treatment of diarrhea, as none of them treats the actual cause.

Constipation

Constipation means infrequent hard stools — less often than every three or four days and hard enough to cause discomfort or pain. Left to himself, that is without you fussing over him, a child will empty his bowel whenever the rectum becomes full. The regularity with which he does this is individual to himself and not to you. Most children manage perfectly well without opening medicines. A diet rich in roughage (fresh fruit and vegetables, bran, cereal, etc.) will encourage regular bowel motions. Constipation without any other signs of illness is really nothing to worry about. Constipation *per se* cannot make a child ill; old theories that constipation could poison the system have long been discarded. Far better than resorting to laxatives is to alter your child's diet slightly to include more roughage, fruit juices and possibly stewed prunes or figs. With very rare exceptions, chronic constipation is almost always due to an overfussy parent who has become obsessive about the regularity of the child's bowel motions.

Mouth Ulcers

The cause of mouth ulcers is known neither in adults nor in children, though we do know some people have a greater tendency than others to get them. A mouth ulcer is exquisitely painful and may be found on the cheeks, the gums or the tongue. When affecting the gums it must not be confused with a gumboil, which is a much larger, redder swelling due to an abcess at the root of the tooth. Mouth ulcers typically come and go in about ten days and there is little we can do to speed up healing. A useful though painful treatment for older children is to rub one or two alum crystals on to the ulcer crater. This makes the ulcer shrink and heal more quickly and helps to reduce subsequent pain. If recurrent mouth ulcers are a problem, it's worth consulting your doctor and obtaining from him a steroid ointment which is put up in a special base that is not dissolved away by saliva.

Teething

Teething should never be blamed as a cause of illness in a baby. Contrary to what you might hear, it does not cause bronchitis, diaper rash, vomiting, diarrhea or loss of appetite. If your baby is irritable and bad-tempered and you can see a tooth coming through his gum, your doctor may prescribe a mild analgesic. Teething jellies that contain local anesthetic have a temporary effect and may cause an allergy. Teething powders are ineffective. You may be fortunate enough to have a child whose teeth erupt without any change in his routine or mood, or you may have a child who becomes miserable as each tooth comes through. In the latter case the best thing to do is to comfort him, distract him, give him a teething ring or a crust of bread or a rusk to bite on. There's no magic remedy.

Infectious Diseases

The common infectious diseases of childhood are nearly all virus illnesses — measles, German measles, chicken pox and mumps — with the exception of whooping cough, which is caused by a bacterium. Babies under the age of six months rarely contract these diseases because they have circulating in their blood antibodies to the diseases that their mother has experienced, these antibodies having crossed the placenta into their bloodstream. Antibodies to whooping cough, however, cross the placenta much less easily than those to

Common Infectious Diseases

	Incubation period	Quarantine	Type of Illness
MEASLES	11 days	10 days from the appearance of the rash	First affects nose and throat and eyes. Fever may reach 39.5 °C (103 °F) and may persist for 6 days. Rash comes out between third and fifth day, starting behind ears. The ears and lungs may become infected later.
GERMAN MEASLES	14–21 days	Unknown	Rash starts behind the ears and lasts for 1–2 days. There is a mild fever of 38.3 °C (101 °F). Enlarged glands appear first at the back of the neck.
WHOOPING COUGH	7–10 days	28 days	The most serious of infectious diseases. In young children there is no 'whoop,' only paroxysms of coughing. Ear and lung infections may occur.
CHICKEN POX	16–17 days	24 hours before the spots appear until all have scabbed	This is a mild illness. Spots come out in crops every 3–4 days and may leave shallow scars.
MUMPS	17–21 days	7 days after the swelling subsides	This is a mild illness and starts with pain, swelling and tenderness of the sides of the face then neck.

Treatment	Return to school	Comments
Darkness is not necessary. There is no specific therapy for the uncomplicated illness other than aspirin. If secondary infection of the ears or lungs supervenes antibiotics are needed.	Any time your child feels like it after 10 days from the appearance of the rash.	Most outbreaks in late winter and early spring. Small white (koplik) spots on the insides of the cheeks clinch the diagnosis.
No specific treatment	When your child is normally active.	Take care not to let pregnant women near your child, as the virus can affect their babies.
Antibiotics must be given early to be effective.	After 28 days when your child is fit.	Specially virulent in babies under one year, so keep your baby away from cases.
Relieve itching with calamine lotion. Treat infected spots with cream from your doctor.	When all the scales have dropped off.	Mainly affects children under ten.
Simple analgesics and lots to drink because the mouth can be dry. Chewing may be painful, so give soft food.	A good week after the swelling goes down.	Not uncommon before the age of five. May be complicated by headache and abdominal pain.

other infectious diseases and this is probably why babies are more susceptible to whooping cough than to the other diseases. This type of immunity is called 'passive immunity' and is fairly short-lived. If you want your baby to be actively immune to certain of the infectious diseases and to be protected against an infection for years, the child must undergo the program of immunization discussed later (see page 128).

The infectious fevers pass easily from one child to another, usually in small droplets of moisture that are breathed out and are circulating in the air. All of the infectious diseases are most infectious just when the first signs of the illness are beginning to show.

The time between catching the disease and developing signs of it is called the incubation period. Quarantine is the length of time that a child should be isolated from other people until he or she becomes noninfectious. Quarantine regulations have been relaxed in recent years, as it is now known that even stringent adherence to them does not prevent the spread of an infectious disease. It is almost impossible to stop one of these infectious fevers from spreading through a family or a closed community like a school because very often the infection has spread even before the illness is diagnosed.

Most of the infectious fevers have a telltale rash which by its character and distribution will implicate one of them. If the appearance of the rash raises your suspicions, don't take your child to the doctor's office, where he may spread it, but telephone the doctor and ask his or her advice. Your description may well enable your doctor to diagnose your baby's illness, and though no treatment may be needed he will tell you how to nurse your child.

How to Nurse Your Child at Home

ACTIVITY

There is absolutely no need to keep sick children in bed. They should be allowed to do what they feel like doing. Those with a high temperature will almost certainly go to bed without your suggesting it. On the other hand, if your child tells you that she would like to get out of bed, she's almost certainly well enough to do so. Neither does she need to be bundled up in an especially warm room. If she wants to lie down she will be happier lying on a couch where she can be near you, and a room temperature that is equable for the rest of the family is suitable for her. You must, however, use your judgment. Sick children will get tired easily and at this point will probably welcome a decision from you that they should go to bed, especially if you or another member of the family is prepared to stay and read to them or play with them for a while.

DIET

Sick children should eat when and what they want. Forcing them to eat will only add to their distress, though drinks should be liberally supplied. An ill child often prefers small, frequent meals and should be given them. Keeping fluid intake up is infinitely more important than maintaining a normal diet. It's good sense to make sure that what your child drinks will nourish her. Fruit juices contain many vitamins, not only vitamin c, and if they are sweet they will provide sugar for energy. Milk, if your child will take it, is of course the best food because it contains protein, minerals, sugar and vitamins. Many children find plain milk unpalatable when they're ill, so give your child a treat and add a fruit flavor. It's quite unnecessary to prepare a special diet and the so-called specially formulated glucose drinks have nothing to offer over plain tap water and white sugar.

TAKING TEMPERATURES

A cool parental hand on the forehead is almost as good an index as any toward diagnosing a fever, but if you wish to be more exact, use a clinical thermometer which can be obtained from any drugstore. Most thermometers, whether they are calibrated on the Fahrenheit or Centigrade scale, will have a normal temperature marked with a small arrow. It is 98.4 on the Fahrenheit scale and 36.6 on the Centigrade scale. Temperatures can be taken by placing the thermometer in the mouth, under the arm or in the rectum. In a small child the safest way to take a temperature is to lay her face down over your knees and to push the thermometer gently into the rectum, holding it firmly between the fingers of your flat hand pressed to her bottom while your other hand holds her shoulders and head still. When a child is old enough to be trusted, a thermometer can be placed under her tongue in her mouth. You must take care not to do this immediately after a hot or a cold drink. The newest thermometers will give you an accurate reading within half a minute. It's irritating for a child to be kept waiting any longer than this.

TREATING A TEMPERATURE

Doctors more often have to tell parents to unwrap their children than instruct them to put on more clothes, so make sure that your're not making your child's temperature worse by having her dressed in too many layers. If your child is well enough to get out of bed, a tepid bath can make her a great deal more comfortable. If she's too ill for this, sponging her with tepid water can bring down her temperature a degree or so. You should not continue tepid sponging when her temperature falls below 39°C (102°F).

MAKING SURE CHILDREN TAKE THEIR MEDICINE

Most medicines nowadays have a pleasant flavor and children enjoy taking them, particularly in the syrup form. If she has to take tablets, help your child by crushing them between two spoons and burying them in jam or some of her favorite food. If your child is taking a course of antibiotics, it's essential that she has her medicine at regular intervals for the prescribed period, so use whatever power you have to cajole her, even proffering candies as rewards.

KEEPING A SICK CHILD OCCUPIED

Most young children need a lot of amusing when they are sick and at home. Your main aim should be to keep them happy, so relax all your rules and allow them to do what they like, even if it means putting a polythene sheet over the bedclothes so that they can paint, even allowing them to play with toys that are 'forbidden,' such as those belonging to the older children. If it isn't too inconvenient, moving the television set into the child's room will do a great deal to improve her spirits. There is no substitute for your company, so do make an effort to read to your child, help her to cut out pictures from old magazines or play a game with her whenever you can. Other members of the family should take their turn at doing this too, knowing that their kindness will be reciprocated when they are ill. Overlook an untidy, messy bedroom.

When your child is not in danger of infecting anyone else, it's a great treat for her to have a visitor, perhaps a neighboring child or a schoolmate. As soon as your child is fit enough to be running around the house, she is fit enough to go outside, and probably fit enough to return to school, although it is worth consulting the principal about this.

Infectious Skin Disorders

COLD SORES

Cold sores have little to do with colds. They are caused by a virus (herpes simplex) that lives permanently in the skin. These viruses are inactive most of the time, but if for any reason the body is heated up, then the virus is activated and a cold sore will result. A high fever or even sitting out in strong sunlight is therefore sufficient to bring out a cold sore. They normally occur around the lips and the cheeks and are very often transmitted from mother to child by kissing. A tingling sensation is felt over the skin where a cold sore is beginning to develop, and if you apply treatment at this time it is possible to abort the development of a cold sore. There are several preparations on the market that can alleviate symptoms of a cold sore, but those that will actually prevent a cold sore from appearing are only available on prescription.

WARTS

Warts are also caused by a virus. They have a natural history of about two years. It takes the body that long to build up antibodies to the virus and so kill it and the wart. This is why old wives' cures sometimes work if well-timed. When I used to supervise a wart clinic, I was always prepared to charm away a wart that had been there for eighteen months or more, usually with some success. Warts are unsightly on the hands and painful on the feet (verrucae). Proprietary wart cures are largely ineffective. There are many now available on prescription which can be used quite safely in the home and achieve a high degree of success. Recalcitrant warts and verrucae will need hospital treatment.

RINGWORM

Ringworm is caused by a fungus that may effect the skin or scalp, causing the typical red circular patch in the skin or bald spots on the scalp. It is quite easy for a doctor to diagnose ringworm: the hairs that are infected with the fungus will fluoresce if placed in ultraviolet light. The treatment for ringworm is simple and sure and free of discomfort. It must be obtained from a doctor.

Allergic Skin Disorders

INFANTILE ECZEMA

Though there is nearly always an allergic element in infantile eczema, it is largely constitutional in origin. In other words it is inherited, and though no other members of your family have eczema they may suffer from remote conditions such as migraine, travel sickness, asthma, or allergies to drugs or foods which are related to eczema. Infantile eczema can start within the first few months of life, and in a young baby is a fairly generalized red, itchy, dry, scaling rash that has a predilection for the face, for the inner sides of the arms and behind the knees. The skin condition has a waxing and waning character, possibly getting worse when the baby has a cold or loses sleep and then clearing when his routine returns to normal. A baby with infantile eczema can be a problem for parents, causing sleepless nights and anxiety. The possibility of skin infections can be a worry especially when a child is confined to diapers. On the optimistic side, some children outgrow their eczema by the age of two and the vast proportion of children are clear by the age of seven. The everyday care of an eczematous skin is fairly simple — meticulous attention to cleanliness, avoidance of overbathing, and frequently rubbing in soft, bland creams and ointments. Further specific treatment should be carried out under the instructions of your doctor. It's necessary that both you and the baby have your sleep, so seek advice from your doctor regarding this.

HIVES (URTICARIA)

Children have a tendency to develop hives which is lost as they grow older. Hives is the only skin condition that disappears completely within minutes and is fairly easy to diagnose. It is very itchy while it lasts but you can do quite a lot to relieve the itch by cooling the skin with applications of calamine lotion. Hives can be caused by foods, by bacteria and viruses and by medicines. One of the commonest offending agents is aspirin, which can bring about not only hives but swelling of the face, eyelids and mouth. Unless attacks of hives are apparent and persistent there is no need for any specific treatment, but they should be investigated to try to find a cause that is removable. A particular form of urticaria named papular urticaria is caused by fleas, usually from the family cat. If a child becomes allergic to flea bites, he may develop spots all over the body which resemble hives but which persist. The cure is to get rid of the fleas or the cat.

Care of the Teeth

The milk teeth are well worth looking after, as teeth lost through decay can cause the permanent teeth to grow crookedly. So all of my boys first visited the dentist at two years old. Tooth decay in most small children is caused by too much sugary food and drink and poor cleaning. Given that children can't escape some sugar and shouldn't be entirely deprived of sweets, I advocate careful brushing with gentle circular movements after sweet foods (make sure the brush is nylon, has unshaped bristles and a flat handle); a fluoride tablet a day from at least two up until twelve years of age; fluoride toothpaste; and six-monthly visits to the dentist.

Immunization

The aim of immunization is to prepare the body to repel infection. Under ordinary circumstances, when a germ enters the body for the first time, the body responds by forming antibodies to that particular germ, or antitoxins that will neutralize the poisons produced by the germ. If the germ attacks you a second time, the body is prepared and can protect itself. By means of an injection (as with measles and diphtheria), or drops by mouth (as with polio) or scratching the skin (as with smallpox), we can help our children to achieve immunity to a number of common childhood infectious diseases. While protection may not be 100 percent, if your child does contract an infection against which he has been immunized, that infection will probably be in a mild form.

An immunization/vaccination scheme is not only for the protection of your baby but also for the good of the community, for when the immunization rate is high the rate of infection is low. As the number of defaulters increases so does the number of cases of infection, so it's vital to take a responsible attitude toward vaccination.

It's quite usual for a small red bump to develop at the site of your baby's injection, but if he develops a fever or becomes irritable get in touch with your doctor. It's important to keep a vaccination

Family Immunization Chart

	NAME	NAME	NAME	NAME
	BORN	BORN	BORN	BORN
DPT (diphtheria, tetanus and pertussis) triple injection at 2, 4, 6, 18 months and preschool	1st	1st	1st	1st
	2nd	2nd	2nd	2nd
	3rd	3rd	3rd	3rd
	4th	4th	4th	4th
	5th	5th	5th	5th
Polio (trivalent oral polio vaccine) at 2, 4, 6, 18 months and preschool	1st	1st	1st	1st
	2nd	2nd	2nd	2nd
	3rd	3rd	3rd	3rd
	4th	4th	4th	4th
	5th	5th	5th	5th

	NAME	NAME	NAME	NAME
	BORN	BORN	BORN	BORN
Measles at 15 months	Date	Date	Date	Date
Rubella (German measles) at 15 months	Date	Date	Date	Date
Mumps at 15 months	Date	Date	Date	Date
Tuberculin skin test	Date	Date	Date	Date

record of dates and types, partly to remind yourself when you need to take your baby for his next dose, and also to help your doctor to complete the program.

The preceding chart is based on recommendations by the American Academy of Pediatrics. Consult your doctor about the specific needs of your child.

10 Developing Personal Relationships

The relationship between caring parent and child is the blueprint for all others. In terms of give and take it's unique. There is no other relationship in which one partner is unconditionally sacrificial, endlessly protective and doggedly loving in the face of the interminably demanding, inconsiderate, egotistical bad-tempered behavior of the other. It is primarily from his parents that a child first meets, then appreciates, then learns and finally responds to all that's best in human behavior. It's the gentler aspects of human behavior that a baby first becomes familiar with. As life is inescapably bound up with forming bonds with other human beings, the sooner he learns that these are more easily made with friendly overtures than hostile approaches the better.

Early Two-Way Communication

Until quite recently, it was thought that babies were unaware of their surroundings until they reacted to them. So for generations babies were offered little stimulation before the age of six weeks. We now know that those first six weeks were almost entirely wasted, for they cover a crucial learning period. Newborn babies are more aware of sights, sounds, and movements than we ever imagined. How we didn't suspect this earlier is a puzzle. It is more than three decades since Konrad Lorenz in his experiments with goslings showed that the sight of the first moving object is imprinted forever in a newborn brain. More than that, the first moving object is indelibly appreciated as the mother figure. Are human babies the same? That we don't know for certain, but there is mounting evidence that they are. Within seconds of birth, some babies will open their eyes, even turn them at the sound of a human voice. I well remember clutching my wet, bluish, newborn second son and whispering his name. His eyes opened and flickered. I had registered! By the end of the first week of life, babies can distinguish their mother's voice, or the voice of the person who undertakes the major part of their care, from all others and will start sucking movements at the sound. Long before their eyes can focus they can perceive shapes, patterns and movements which will make their hearts beat faster without any change of expression registering on their faces.

What does all this mean? It means it's never too early to start treating your baby (let's say it's a boy) as another human being with a character and personality of his own which you can help shape — shape in the best possible sense by showing that the currency of human relationships is love, gentleness, reciprocity, encouragement, delight. . . . Your baby will learn surprisingly quickly. At first he wants nothing more than to be dry, warm and well fed. Following on from this he very quickly wants your approbation. He sees you smile and interprets this as friendship. He wishes to be friendly back. Your baby smiles. You smile more, you kiss him, hug him. He enjoys that. He smiles more to please you so that you will do the things that please him. It's his first attempt at two-way conversation and, though you probably hadn't realized it, he's taken the initiative. Learning to smile for his parents and then later for others is a very important skill to learn. It's a friendly approach to another person. Such an approach is nearly always greeted joyfully and the habit in your baby is reinforced. Hopefully it is one he will always keep. If you smile back encouragingly at your baby from the beginning, you will be helping to make your child into an outgoing, friendly person.

Facial contact is also important. Research has shown that parents who face their children while feeding or playing and look into their eyes are less likely to smack their children as they grow up and are more likely to be sympathetic arbitrators. Not surprisingly the children of such parents are better able to form relationships with others as they get older, for despite ourselves we invariably distrust the shifty eyed. Children are equally, if not more, sensitive to the eye that will not meet theirs and quite often will admonish a parent with, ''Mummy, *look* at me.''

In the early months babies use crying as the only language with which to make requests, expecting and hoping that their request will be met. If their cry for help is answered they gradually learn how demands are made and that other human beings will respond to any reasonable demand reasonably made. In other words, they begin to appreciate the basic give and take of a relationship. If a baby's requests go unanswered he quickly learns there's no point in making them and that those people nearest him don't try to help. The baby is encouraged to grow up self-contained, uncommunicative and unkind. This is why I am wholeheartedly against letting babies cry themselves to sleep and distrust parents who say, "He needs to cry for half an hour to exercise his lungs," or, "She used to cry a lot but she's as good as gold now." You need never be afraid to lavish love on your baby. Under the age of one year a baby cannot be spoiled. He will accept all the affection you can give him like a sponge and be all the better for it.

Relationships within the Family

Once a baby has learned the basic patterns of behavior with his mother and father he then tries them out within the family group. Recently the idea of the family has come under attack from psychologists and others. While acknowledging that families are not all good and a bad one may inflict lasting damage, I'm convinced there's nothing to beat a good one. I see a family as an extended group, fundamentally stable, encompassing strong and lasting relationships, in which a child can grow up feeling secure and well loved, to which he must contribute, and in which his voice is heard.

I consider it important that a child becomes able to relate to people of all ages. Though he may prefer to spend most of his time with children of his own age, he should meet relatives and friends who are older. While at first they may be his parents' friends, he should learn that they are automatically his, too. Friends come in all ages, sizes and colors. Friends can help children to become socially unafraid. Though perhaps frightened at first, children must learn to relate to strangers, and it's easiest and most comfortable if they start to do this within the safe, familiar surroundings of home. Friends and relatives may serve to modify the effect of the nuclear family by relieving tensions and broadening horizons.

Grandparents have a very important role to play in helping a child to develop his personality and can be very valuable assets to a family. By virtue of their age they are generally philosophical, long-suffering and sympathetic in their dealings with grandchildren. The best grandparents interpret warning signs and anticipate problems and head them off. They pacify by distraction, not by insistence, and so obtain obedience quite readily. Free from the direct responsibility of bringing up the children, grandparents will more often than not have the time and inclination to persuade with patience and have learned the knack of understanding and handling children with ease. It is said that grandparents spoil their grandchildren. In many cases this is misuse of the word *spoil*. If spoiling a child means giving explanations instead of dismissals, suggesting alternatives instead of negatives, and helping instead of ignoring, then grandparents do spoil children. The presence of grandparents in the house can often be a boon to the family and given that they don't cause friction with the parents they should be welcomed.

Confidence through Encouragement

It has been known for years that the best system of bringing up children is the one that lays emphasis on encouragement and reward. For instance, children in the care of institutions run by kind, loving housemothers gain more weight than those who are cared for by strict disciplinarians. And it isn't only children who respond to love and care. Adults praised for good work can manage a higher output than a group who are kept strictly in line and punished for misdemeanors. There is no human being who is worse off for being shown kindness and affection. The need for affection, encouragement and reward in children is acute and they should be overtly praised whenever they are good or do something well. A useful rule is to tell your child you love her at least once a day, and as often as you like. In addition to building up a loving relationship, you build confidence, self-assurance and security in your child and will start teaching her praiseworthy qualities and the boundaries of civil behavior to others.

The Right Atmosphere

Keeping yourself happy is an important ingredient in maintaining a good relationship with your child. You will notice that you get on better with everyone, including your family, if your own life is going well. Children are rapidly affected by what is going on around them. As a rule happy, outgoing parents will find they have a happy, outgoing child. Depressed, short-tempered parents will recognize their own image in their child. Maladjusted parents will breed maladjustment in the home, with maladjusted children who, never having experienced a good relationship with their parents, fail to manage it with others.

The head start provided by a good home will carry a child well into later life to the time when she starts to make her own personal ground rules for behavior; one hopes it will smooth the way through her first exposure to a group of complete strangers.

Introduction to Nursery School

Most children want to start mixing with larger groups at about the age of two and a half or three, and a friendly nursery school, if you want to send your child to one, can do much to fulfill this need. The aim of nursery schools and playgroups is not just to widen a child's learning experiences beyond the home, but to encourage sociability which should also grow beyond the family circle. Choosing the right nursery school is a serious business. You are turning your child over to others for almost half of his waking day and it requires a good deal of objective research on your part.

Research means visiting the nursery schools with your child, meeting the teachers, and sitting in on the nursery class. You'll find that most good nursery schoolteachers welcome your interest and don't view it with suspicion. Having decided on a school, you must do all you can to help your child settle in happily. In the beginning this may mean keeping your child company for the whole morning, possibly during the first week or so until he will allow you to go, say, after an hour. At first leave him for only half an hour, with the excuse that you have an errand to do. Be sure to return when you promised, so that the child feels he can rely on you coming back. Gradually he'll need you less and less. Eventually he will run to join his friends as soon as he gets to school and say goodbye to you quite happily. This process of adjustment to school should not be rushed beyond the child's natural inclination. You must be prepared to go slowly and if necessary retrace a step or two if something upsets him. A child must never be pushed into school against his will. He will not only interpret it as an unkind act and resent you — and possibly the teachers too — but he may permanently regard school as an unpleasant place, and this will slow down his learning.

All of my three sons presently at school were happier if I stayed with them for the first few minutes of each morning, up to the age of five. The eldest was happy and reassured if we'd started a jigsaw puzzle together and he had something to work on after I left. The second would immediately present me with paper and crayons and we'd draw a picture together. The third still likes me to take off his coat, go with him to the classroom and wave to him from the school gate, so I do because I don't want him to associate going to school with the unhappiness of a perfunctory farewell.

Answering Children's Questions

Most mothers start talking to their babies within a few minutes of birth because they are driven to verbalize the love they feel. What we sometimes forget is that we should keep on talking, keep on verbalizing that love. Children who are spoken to often learn the mechanics of communication more readily. Children who are encouraged to converse learn the use of language more quickly. Most important, children who are encouraged to question, who are given explanations, who take for granted that parents will listen to them, however halting their speech, are not only happier children but grow up much less authoritarian than those whose questions are ignored, who are rarely supplied with explanations (particularly for dos and donts that are blindly enforced) and who are hardly ever considered as individuals with something to say.

Questions should never be avoided even if they embarrass you. When do you tell your child about sex? The first time he asks you. But remember, telling the truth does not necessarily mean explaining everything. A child's curiosity should always be matched by your willingness to answer truthfully. And it is surely better that he learns about sex in an accurate matter-of-fact way from you than in a secretive melodramatic way from his friends. In his early years your child will regard you as omniscient and will naturally turn to you for advice on all subjects. If you remain approachable and welcome questions he will grow up feeling he can talk to you about anything. Discouraging children when they are young and uninhibited will do little to lessen their inhibitions as they grow older. If you are determined that you will always remain the ready confidante of your children it is worth keeping the channels of communication open, no matter what it costs you.

Children's sex education begins with their first cuddle. They take pleasure in physical contact and joy in their parents' reciprocity, and will grow up realizing that people touch one another as an act of friendship as well as of love. As they get older they will become pleasantly aware of their bodies without being self-conscious about them. This can be encouraged by an open attitude to nudity within the family — if you have no objection. A child who sees his parents unclothed as a matter of course is unlikely to be concerned about his own nakedness. On the other hand, if you are worried about it, your child will almost certainly worry too. Curiosity about his mother's breasts and his father's penis is best satisfied by a frank chat and a good look, neither of which is likely to stimulate sexual feelings.

Babies become aware of their genital organs by the end of the first year and frequently handle them without any obvious pleasure. There'll come a day however, when it does bring a pleasurable sensation, and their fondling becomes more like real masturbation. Nearly all children of both sexes masturbate. It is perfectly normal and will not lead to blindness, homosexuality, insanity or any of the other fictitious penalties. Unless it is an obsessional means of escaping from reality, the best way to treat it is by paying no attention. If it happens in public, distraction is the best course, but never scold. This will only encourage anxiety and furtiveness and increase the child's desire to masturbate. Children usually indulge in frequent masturbation only if another part of their life is empty. In treating that cause you must look to yourself. (See section on masturbation on page 88).

Children first inquire about death when they are old enough to grow fond of someone and therefore to fear losing him. This may be prompted by a death in the family or the death of a pet or just by seeing a dead bird in the garden. Permanent absence is a difficult and painful concept for a child to grasp, and usually cannot be accepted before the age of eight. In explaining death it's best not to use words like *sleep* because then your child may become afraid of going to sleep, or *taken* because he may suspect that he will be taken in the same way. All questions about death should be answered truthfully. You cannot protect your child from death; you can only help him to come to terms with the idea that everyone and everything (including leaves and flowers) dies eventually. So if your child asks you outright, ''Will Granny ever come back?'' don't shield him, say ''No.'' If he gets worried about dying himself it will not help at all if you answer that death only happens to old people like Granny. It's better to be realistic and say that he may, but as it's so unlikely it's not worth worrying about.

11 Learning

Stimulus and Praise

Babies start to learn with their first feeding, be it on the bottle or on the breast. The breast soon becomes a malleable plaything through which the baby learns to explore and experiment. She strokes and kneads it and quickly learns that her handling stimulates the let-down reflex of milk, making feeding easier. By using her hands the baby finds that the resilient, comforting nature of the breast can introduce her to pleasurable sensations. Learning to manipulate a bottle is an equally important process as the bottle soon becomes a toy. It's obvious that most babies enjoy feeding not only because it satisfies their appetite but also because they enjoy the fun and play that goes along with the whole routine. If you bottle feed your baby try to incorporate relaxed gentle play periods into feeding times. For the first few years of life children do much of their learning through play. In fact play can be said to be the key to learning. No child has to be taught to play, so in a young child learning should be synonymous with play. It follows that the transition from activities by which the child is learning through playing to those by which she's learning through working should be imperceptible. And it can all start with feeding.

At first you are your child's plaything, her main companion, her only toy. It is not just more fun for both of you if you respond to the baby's games — you will have the satisfaction of teaching new skills, widening her experience, introducing her to language, and stimulating her curiosity. So you should respond whenever the spirit takes you and talk, sing, recite rhymes to your baby, play games with her and give her a cuddle any time at all. Children enjoy being chatted to and appreciate rhythmic songs or clapping games long before you'd ever think. They absorb what they need and what they enjoy from any game and discard the rest. You need not worry about their not understanding or about your seeming ridiculous. If they see you playing games they are more likely to start imitating you (not necessarily accurately, but that doesn't matter), which is one of the first steps in learning to learn. As babies gain courage they will try to join in and start learning to participate in games. They will do this all the more readily if you praise their every achievement and encourage all their endeavors. We all know the satisfaction of praise; and small children actually *need* it. Their pleasure at being praised is radiant and we should lavish that praise unstintingly. Praise, praise, praise — there's absolutely no substitute.

Responding to your baby does not only mean passively applauding her efforts. It means observing her own individual needs and taking part in as many of her various activities as you can manage. In the early years these activities nearly always happen right under your feet. Small children want to be with you and some devoted parents, in order to share their presence and time with their children, have been known to get down and peel the potatoes on the floor or get into the playpen beside their children! Responsive parents will always encourage curiosity, experimentation and adventurousness, qualities that make learning not only more interesting but more rewarding. From a surprisingly early age you can encourage your child to be observant and to concentrate. She will be happy to study a mobile over her crib for long periods. The bare ceiling holds no such charm. By placing her carriage under a tree you give her the changing patterns of the wind on the leaves to look at. As early as a month old, babies can safely be propped up so that they can take an interest in what's going on around them. Besides widening their horizons all these things are teaching them to be contented and independent.

Progress and Development: Critical Phases

While we know that a baby may start learning very soon after he's born, we know that the rate of learning isn't constant. There are learning peaks when the baby seems to be able to develop new skills with great ease, absorb information very quickly and put new experiences to immediate use. No two children have learning peaks at the same age. It's better to respond to the progress of your own child than to check him off against development charts. Learning peaks may last weeks or months when children may take extraordinary leaps forward. During these spurts it's vital that you are especially helpful to your child and devote to him all the time and attention you can spare, though one or two hours of concentrated work/play with your child is probably better than a whole day of half-hearted tolerance of his demands.

It may be that children not only pass through phases when they learn quickly. There may be periods when parts of their brains associated with special skills come to maturity. Unless that special skill is introduced at that time the receptive phase passes and the skill can never be properly learned. There are examples in the animal kingdom. If baby birds are reared in complete silence up to the age of eight weeks they will never learn to sing, even though they're exposed to birdsong later. Other experiments have shown that kittens kept in darkness beyond their sixth week never learn to see, even though the rest of their life is spent in daylight. This evidence would seem to suggest that for baby birds a trigger that sets off the desire and ability to communicate occurs at about eight weeks and for kittens the coming together of all the different aspects of brain function that allow sight happens at six weeks. It is frightening that the capability is retained for such a short time; it is salutary that it appears so early in life. It is unlikely that human babies develop on the same time scale; nonetheless the evidence for relatively short aptitude peaks is of long standing.

In 1890 William James stated the law of transitoriness, which concerns the waxing and waning nature of instincts.

> If during the time of an instinct's vivacity, the objects adequate to arouse it are met with, a habit of acting on them is formed, which remains when the original instinct has passed away; but if no such objects are met with, then no habit will be formed; and later on in life when the animal meets the objects he will altogether fail to react, as at an earlier epoch he would instinctively have done.*

This theory has led us today to the concept of the 'critical phase' in childhood development, which states that if the proper or necessary environment stimulus does not appear at the time of emergence of a

---

* Lois Barclay Murphy Associates, *The Widening World of Childhood* (New York: Basic Books, 1962), p. 307.

new function, the function will not develop when it should and will never develop thereafter.

We now know that the development of centers in the brain associated with learning can only take place during the first years of life, and a child's capability for learning is complete before school entry. There is very convincing evidence that the patterns of brain activity for learning processes, e.g. memory, judgment, decision making, problem solving, planning ahead, being methodical, giving attention to detail, powers of concentration, have been laid down in the first five years for the rest of life. This means it falls largely to parents to provide for their children the necessary stimuli that favor the development of emerging skills. Research shows that your child can't have two bites at the cherry and most skills emerge before school age. It's a weighty responsibility for parents. What teachers do is minuscule in comparison.

This does not mean that children should ever be pushed hard when they're young. It may turn a child off reading for ever to be forced to learn with flash cards for tedious weeks when he would have done as well in a few hours only a year later. To a child, writing and drawing are natural extensions of scribbling, but it would be quite wrong for you to force this refinement on him. You must wait for your child's lead. He'll give you a clear signal when he wishes to graduate. Infinitely more important is to give him the help he asks for when he's ready.

The Value of Play

As far as a baby or a child is concerned, play is learning is work. Adults make semantic distinctions, such as play is fun/work is serious/work cannot be fun/work cannot be play. Children make no such distinction. While for adults the word *play* has connotations of idleness and unproductiveness, for children play is very hard work. It isn't that children are too young to work, but that playing is just about their only form of work. And while they're playing they're growing up and learning.

Here are some of the ways that play helps learning:

1. Play helps children to get to know themselves. Before they can hope to integrate themselves with others they

have to understand themselves. Play allows them to find their physical and intellectual strengths and weaknesses.

2. Play puts the world around them into perspective. A game such as a farmyard with animals can introduce them to aspects of life their own immediate experience would omit, at the same time reducing the world to a scale that they can literally handle and maneuver.

3. Play can develop, or be an outlet for, emotions. Giving a boy a doll can bring out feelings of protectiveness and gentleness that were dormant. Using the same toy the child can give reign to aggressive instincts that if directed against people could be antisocial.

4. Play can create an interest in people. A dressing-up box with cowboy outfits and nurses' uniforms can help to make children interested in people from different walks of life — what do people do, and what is needed to do it — and understand that in later life most people do a job of work.

5. Play can increase a child's ability to communicate. Social play encourages a mastery of language that goes beyond simple demands. The more imaginative the play, the more complex the ideas that need to be expressed in terms that others understand.

6. Play helps physical coordination. Freedom to climb, swing, skip, run and jump helps to perfect muscular movement and physical skills, while also improving vision and hearing.

7. Play can improve normal dexterity. Doing even a simple jigsaw or building a tower of bricks helps children to get used to making their hands work for them as tools, until they can graduate to more taxing exercises posed by handicraft and mechanical toys.

8. Play can develop the senses of territory and ownership. The importance of a new and highly cherished toy or their own private place to play, their 'camp,' can teach children to respect the belongings and privacy of others.

9. Play with friends can teach a child to get along with others. Having friends to the house as soon as your child becomes sociable helps to teach him to overcome shyness, to be prepared to share, to work out small problems without adult intervention, and to control outbursts of emo-

tional behavior. Your child may find a special friend and learn to love, to understand problems to do with feelings that he can't easily verbalize, and to consider the wishes of others.

10. Play can stimulate curiosity, independence, an open adventurous spirit and intellectual growth. You can stimulate your child's intellectual activity by his surroundings as well as by play. Coloring the room yellow or blue has been proved to make a child brighter. Toys that fit shapes into appropriate holes stimulate analytical thought and help intellectual growth. As your child gets older, toys that allow experimentation like a microscope, a telescope, a chemistry set, a magician's outfit, teach how to meet challenges and master difficulties.

11. Play can help children to learn to cope. The loss of a treasured toy or friend, the failure to make a mechanical toy work, the frustration of having desires that exceed competence, the difficulty of several choices, managing the pain of falling off a bicycle, the decision to go out or stay at home all help children to learn to cope with problems that arise in their environment.

12. Play helps children to mature. As early as the age of three they may show signs of a *planning* sense. For instance, that traffic jam of toy cars under surveillance by a police car and helped by a pickup truck shows that they're thinking ahead. They will increase their *capacity to delay* by playing with toys that need the glue to set or the clay to dry. Sharing one of their toys with a friend who reciprocates can teach them the value of *manipulating the environment*.

Creative Play

Activities that involve creative play are especially beneficial to children. They are a treasure trail of discovery and delight. Creative games that need no supervision allow children to follow any interesting development as the fancy takes them so that they can concentrate on doing something of their own choosing, using their own judgment to the complete fulfillment of their interest. Such games quite often require you to turn a blind eye to disorder, even to minor damage, but it's worth it. For instance, once you've resigned yourself to having to wash all your baby's clothes it's a thrill to see her experimenting to her heart's content with soil, trowel and pots while you get on with your gardening. It is mutually beneficial. Your child is experiencing the feel of soil, how she can handle it, what can be done with it, and you're left free to get on with your weeding.

From the age of eighteen months onwards, there's nothing a child enjoys more than to be given the freedom of the kitchen sink and to be allowed to play water games with all the paraphernalia that you can muster. All my sons have spent hours at the taps, sleeves rolled up, almost smothered in an apron, banked round by chairs and cushions so that they can't fall, splashing and pouring for hours. Forget the mess and the fact that the floor is awash and do a massive clearing operation with towels when your child gets bored and wants to move on. It's very good for the child if you can manage to ignore the mess or alternatively take precautions against it spoiling your home. Putting a sheet of polythene on the carpet prevents the Plasticine or play-dough from getting trodden in.

In the summer let your child take his clay or hammer and nails outside. There he can pursue experiments to his heart's content, and his excitement can build without interruption. Simultaneously he's learning how to take on a project and work at it until it's finished. If children are constantly interrupted and told to be clean, tidy and careful, their interest wanes. They lose sight of their end point and become disheartened. This is the sort of treatment that results in children lacking the ability to concentrate when they get to school.

TAKING PART IN HOUSEHOLD CHORES

There are a few activities that are guaranteed to make a child feel useful and therefore cooperative and keen to expand his skills. Being allowed to help in the house is certainly one of them. The child is even happier if his help is actively sought. He feels his contribution is important to you and the family. As soon as children start to toddle they will try to help with all sorts of household chores; without prompting they will heave on the vacuum cleaner, struggle with a dustpan and brush and occasionally rush off for a cloth to mop up spillage. A child given this sort of freedom is more likely to grow up thoughtful and cooperative, ready to do his share and eager to give a helping hand with any project. It encourages him to be independent and self-assured and grow up with the idea that he's needed. This is a great boost to anyone's morale but is especially valuable to a child.

As a child gets older he should be encouraged to help with less pleasant tasks like clearing away the toys, tidying his bedroom, helping with the dishes. One hopes he will take for granted that groups of people interact as a team, and in time of need it's all hands to the wheel. Many children love cooking. When they're four or five they may want to make up imaginary dishes with strange ingredients. As they reach seven or eight they like to follow recipes and make dishes that all the family can eat. Whether it's a dish of pure fantasy or a proper meal, many children see cooking as an interesting and truly creative pastime. As they reach their teens you reap the benefits of your years of patience when your son or daughter offers to make and actually does produce a three-course meal.

Intellectual Skills

The learning of complex intellectual skills like talking, reading, or understanding numbers usually happens piecemeal, with the child retaining odd pieces of information that may take a fairly long time to acquire. So a child of four may recognize the words of her name and read them, even write them, but full competence does not come until she's six or more.

Research has shown that a child uses all available intellectual resources to focus on learning a complex skill. So you can help your child by giving her as many different kinds of aids as possible. Not surprisingly the skill is more readily learned if it is used frequently. A child is exposed to words more often than numbers, and number skills may lag behind word skills. In learning to read, for example, a child puts together many different kinds of information as she learns to recognize word shapes and sounds and to fit words with objects. Like any other person she relies greatly on memory and experience. So a frequently used word slots into her memory earlier and gains meaning more quickly than one she meets rarely. Lessons that are reinforced are recalled more easily than those only met with once. In reading as well as speaking, repetition is very important, so you should try to use a new word as often as possible.

Your child will eventually come to associate words with objects by using her eyes and common sense. The word *Cornflakes* is, not surprisingly, written on a cornflakes box — children quickly latch on to such clues. If taken into a shop and asked, "Where is the counter labeled 'Shoes,'" the average seven-year-old will spot the word *shoes,* even though she's never met it before, by identifying lots of shoes on stands, seeing the word displayed above them and putting two and two together. It follows that a child's reading will benefit from being presented with word-picture or word-object associations.

As she's learning to read from a page your child will quite probably ignore difficult words, and complete sentences not as written but as she thinks they should be completed. Sometimes she will substitute words that look similar but have a different meaning, for example *play* and *plan.* It doesn't really matter as long as your child enjoys reading and is making her own sense of it. It's wrong to interrupt and correct small errors when children are beginning to read. They will correct these errors themselves with usage. It's more important for them to learn word patterns and sentence construction and enjoy gathering information for themselves. So if they hesitate over a word, even the same word repeatedly, say it for them straight away to keep the sense going.

READING

The child's reading material need not be restricted. There is nothing innately good in a children's encyclopedia or innately bad in comic books. Reading should be fun. If you debar frivolous reading matter your child will feel reading is a dry, uninteresting activity and will shrink from it. The important thing is that he reads. As he gets older he can make it as serious as he likes.

While it's important to encourage reading because it can increase a child's world almost more than any other pastime, an undue emphasis on books is not always in every child's best interest. Children who are slow to read but who love to make things with their hands are not necessarily less intelligent and may be more interesting than those who shut themselves away in books. The doer should never be considered inferior to the thinker. Each can learn equally well from his experience and expand his own particular universe. As long as your child sees that books are cherished in your house, he won't pass up the chance to participate in the fun. He'll read in his own good time.

12 Behavior Problems

Causes and Prevention

Though it may be hard for parents to accept, behavior problems in their children nearly always arise because of behavior problems in themselves. An aggressive or jealous or destructive or deceitful child of preschool age is nearly always expressing dissatisfaction with conditions inside the home. The danger is that, unless corrected, the pattern of behavior may become set so that the child will have difficulties at school, then at work, and later in marriage and with his own children and on throughout life. A child with a behavior problem is usually the subject of one of the following:

1. Insecurity
2. The need for comfort
3. The need for affection
4. Overdiscipline
5. Parental conflict
6. Parental ignorance of what is normal child behavior

Nearly all of these conditions arise from three main causes (which in their turn may lead to secondary causes): a poor relationship between the parents; expecting too much too soon from your child, and an unrealistic attitude to discipline. Behavior problems are rare in the children of couples who are loving to one another and are seen by their children to be kind, thoughtful and considerate of each other. It follows, more often than not, that a couple who are devoted to one another will put a great deal of effort into creating a home filled with happiness. They will avoid conflict, particularly where it may affect the children, e.g. over methods of punishment. They will make sure that they don't demand too much from their children; they will breed an atmosphere of permanence, stability and security; they will be openly affectionate. They will build up a sub-

149

stantial credit balance of understanding, reasonableness and fairness with their children.

Discipline

The same parents will take a rational view of discipline. Overdiscipline and underdiscipline can be equally bad for children — both lead to insecurity. Ruling by fear, force, corporal punishment and humiliation never worked for adults, so why should it work for children? On the other hand, offering no guidance at all really serves your child badly, as you only make life harder for her than it need be. Other children, let alone other adults, are not going to tolerate an ill-mannered, selfish bully. There have to be some rules in a home as in any other organized group of people, for the sake of efficiency, justice and safety. Sensible, loving parents, however, keep their rules to a minimum and retain only those that have good reason to support them. Children are interested in and can understand motivation much earlier than you imagine and will appreciate reasons for doing certain things if all is explained simply. They are much more likely to comply with your requests if they understand why you make them. One simple example is bedtimes. There is a persuasive school of thought that advocates a fairly inflexible bedtime routine with a kind but no-nonsense approach, a resistance to delaying tactics, and a firm attitude to crying at bedtime or during the night, refusal to lie down, and requests to come into Mummy's bed. Most children will accept this routine in time even if there are difficulties initially. Most children will also return to it if it is interrupted by an illness or a vacation. This fairly rigid routine is probably fine for a baby who has had one or both of her parents at home most of the day — and almost a necessity for those parents who have their child to cope with all day. As your child gets older she will appreciate the fact that you need a rest and time on your own. If you have to leave your child regularly for a large part of each day, as you will if you work, and there is no good reason why she should go to bed other than that it suits your convenience, she's unlikely to accept a strict bedtime routine without trouble. You cannot reason with a child of less than two and a half or three, so if she is not sleepy, depriving her of your company will only make her unhappy. There is nothing sadder than the idea of children crying themselves to sleep. So when they're small what's to be lost except some of your privacy and serenity if you let them toddle about until they drop. Most children, you will find, actually go to sleep at the same time whether banished to their bedroom or allowed to stay with you. I would advocate the latter; your child acknowledges your love and desire to be with her, and it will be useful on a future occasion when you may need to be stricter. As children get older you can explain to them that you as adults deserve privacy just as they enjoy time to themselves, and they'll accept the idea of playing in their bedroom even though they don't feel ready for sleep.

Punishment

As far as punishment is concerned, unless it is very severe the type of punishment is less important than the spirit in which it is given. A sharp smack given in a flash of anger will do little harm if a child usually enjoys a loving sympathetic relationship with his parents and such punishment is forgotten quickly. It will leave no scar. In fact it may do more good than a long explanatory diatribe, for it may have the desired effect and clear the air immediately. If, on the other hand, a child does not enjoy an affectionate relationship with his parents, he will interpret every smack as proof of their lovelessness. Smacking as a cold, calculated act will always be seen by a child as the cruel act it is. Though disciplinarians find it hard to believe, children who are rarely smacked respond with contrition to a change in tone of voice or facial expression by their parents. Just as continual smacking ceases to have effect, a bad-tempered shout from a habitual shouter goes unheeded. Bearing a grudge is never anything but uncharitable. Don't wait for your child to make it up. Always be the first to offer the olive branch. A child may be afraid to approach you and whereas fifteen minutes to you is a short time, to a child newly punished it may seem an eternity. Each succeeding minute makes him feel more unloved and neglected. Children have a different sense of time from adults.

Bed-wetting

No child under the age of four who still occasionally wets the bed or has accidents during the day should be considered to be backward.

In fact one in ten boys still wets the bed at the age of five. Children develop skills at different rates — this applies particularly to bladder capacity (see Chapter 8). One of the characteristics of bladder control is the ability to hold urine for longer and longer periods. But it may take some children a very long time to develop the capability to last out the ten or so hours through the night. So a child should not be labeled as a bed-wetter when he's still training his bladder up to full capacity. And you can help him with this. You can discourage drinks after 6 P.M. You can make certain your child empties his bladder before going to bed. You can toilet him before you go to bed. You can put a potty by his bed should he wake and want to pass urine. Most children do not have full control of urgency until they're quite old. If they wake wanting to go to the bathroom they'll probably lie there and do it rather than face the journey in the dark, whereas reaching for a potty at the bedside will seem a comparatively easy maneuver.

Habitual bed-wetting after the age of five is called nocturnal enuresis and may benefit from medical advice, but not necessarily. It is nearly always the sign of increased tension and anxiety and classically gets worse just before exams or an important school football game, for instance. In looking for causes, however, it's essential that you examine your own behavior. You may be the source of tension by pushing your child too hard, or by discussing financial troubles in his presence. And if this is the case the bed-wetting won't disappear until you put your own house in order.

As worry and anxiety are the root cause of the problem it seems to me illogical, not to say unkind, to subject your child to anything that may aggravate his sense of inadequacy. Dragging him from doctor to doctor will do this. Using bells and buzzers to waken him when he first starts to pass urine will do this. Trying one kind of drug after another will do this. Only a few of these methods have been shown to have a significant success rate anyway and must be carefully chosen by a pediatrician. I strongly believe that the problem should be minimized, should be accepted by the household as normal and the strain taken off yourself and your child by simple rearrangements of routine. A rubber sheet covered by a small top sheet that can be washed and dried every day if necessary cuts down on washing and smell. Most households can afford some kind of washing machine, but for the household with a bed-wetter it becomes a necessity. And bite your tongue off before you ever scold your child about bed-wetting. No matter how tiresome it becomes, make light of it and change the subject. It's cold comfort, but where do all the bed-wetters go? They grow out of it of course, usually before the age of ten, often *despite* treatment.

Head-Banging and Rocking Movements

Young children usually feel compelled to rock themselves rhythmically because they feel deprived of that same rocking movement that they should experience in their parent's arms, in a swinging cradle or a gently bouncing carriage. For nine months they have jogged and swayed inside their mothers' abdomen. They have been programed to a life that is hardly ever still, so it's not surprising that they feel unhappy when the movement stops. Even being carried around is often sufficient. Some children, if left to lie still for long periods, will try to comfort themselves with rocking movements as soon as they are physically strong enough to do them, which is rarely before five or six months. Then they may start rolling from side to side, banging one side of their head against the crib, or making very strenuous movements in which they lift the whole top half of their bodies almost upright and bring their heads down. It's a warning sign that should be taken seriously because it means the child has been starved of comfort and physical contact in the earliest months. It should be corrected at all costs or the child may grow up expecting affection from no one, looking only to himself for comfort and becoming a loner in the process. To emphasize how important the early months are, head banging, once established, may be impossible to stop, which is certainly detrimental to the child and sometimes to others. Children not only waste valuable time and energy which could be spent widening their learning experience, but they may create enough disturbance to keep awake other children who share the same bedroom.

Nightmares

True nightmares rarely occur before the age of three, though sometimes younger babies wake with a scream and a frightened look that suggests they've had a bad dream. Most children have occasional nightmares that are normal but can be quite frightening if a child doesn't immediately come to, appears not to hear or know you, and expresses her fears in garbled language. Nightmares are not abnormal unless they occur night after night or are accompanied by sleepwalking, which suggests that the child is having to exercise great self-control to overcome her anxieties when she's awake but loses this control when she's asleep. The treatment is to find the cause of the tension and remove it. If the cause is not obvious, talking things over with your doctor may help; he may recommend deeper exploration of the problem by a child psychotherapist.

Thumb-Sucking, Nail-Biting, 'Security Blankets'

None of these is any way abnormal in a young child and no attempt should be made to stop them, especially by forced deprivation or ridicule. A child likes to suck his thumb because sucking is a pleasurable sensation from a very early age. The first time he puts his fingers or his whole fist into his mouth he's exploring an important pleasure-giving part of the body, so thumb-sucking is part of learning about his own body. The fact that it continues when he's bored, concentrating, tired or afraid is of no consequence. Even adults occupy themselves at similar times with similar distractions. Some people who confess to disliking the taste of tobacco nonetheless reach for a cigarette when under stress and make sucking movements.

Nail-biting, though uncommon in preschool children, occurs in about half of otherwise quite normal schoolchildren, and for the most part is an unconscious nervous habit that is best cured by encouraging a pride in appearance — for instance, allowing girls to paint their nails with colorless polish. Most children stop nail-biting when they become concerned about their appearance *vis-à-vis* the opposite sex or reach the age when social considerations outweigh personal habits.

Just as many children who are well loved and come from happy homes have 'security blankets' as those who come from less fortunate backgrounds, so it is not a sign of insecurity or lack of love. Your child should be allowed to take his everywhere until he voluntarily leaves it behind, though sometimes reserving it as a bedtime comfort — even after marriage.

154

Aggressiveness, Destructiveness, Bullying

All of these modes of behavior represent cries for help. They can result from parental absence, parental neglect, overdiscipline, underdiscipline, too much smacking, or parental disharmony. The child herself is really not at fault, though she may seem resistant to offers of help. Curing her of this abnormal behavior and distrust of adults may take years, not months, of relearning by endlessly patient helpers who, because of parental inadequacy, may be teachers, social workers and psychologists. Nasty little children are nearly always nasty because someone has been nasty to them. Don't blame them, look beyond them to their environment.

Lying and Stealing

All children tell the odd fib, often because it's fun to fantasize or to fool another child or especially an adult. Living in a complete fantasy world of lies means that the child is trying to avoid something very unpleasant in his real world, like believing his parents don't love him or being the subject of abuse at school. Such causes should be investigated and corrected. Lying continually to avoid blame stems only from one thing — fear. That means an authority figure in the child's life is using painful threats or, worse still, physical beating or separation as punishment. Lying will not stop until the child learns that telling the truth is more comfortable than telling a lie. It seems to me very understandable that a child should protect his obvious vulnerability with a lie. There's nothing in a child's life that makes truthfulness an attractive proposition in itself, not unless a thoughtful adult purposely makes it so. In our house truthfulness is rewarded, even though it involves a confession to a wrongdoing. The two acts are separated. The children know that telling the truth is highly prized, but that this does not exonerate them from responsibility for their misdemeanor.

Stealing in a young child is nearly always an affection- or attention-seeking device, and again is usually a symptom of too little love in a child's life.

Temper Tantrums and Breath-Holding Attacks

During the years from two to four, temper tantrums must come under the heading of normal. Children of this age have not yet acquired the judgment to match their will and so clashes with parents may be frequent, culminating in a tantrum when the child may throw herself on the floor kicking and screaming because she cannot help herself. A few dos and donts. Do try to stay calm — your child may catch your mood. Do ignore her and leave her on her own — a tantrum loses most of its point if there's no audience. Don't punish her — this will only make things worse. Don't shut the door on her or go far away — let her see where you are so that she doesn't feel deserted, and leave her the option of making it up with you. As she gets older your child will get better at tolerating delays and accepting compromises and you will get more expert at anticipating problems and forestalling head-on clashes by judicious distraction tactics.

Breath-holding attacks are really just extensions of temper tantrums in usually bright children who are stronger willed than average and react very angrily when thwarted. These attacks are usually directed at particularly infuriating incidents. They rarely occur without an audience, and especially not if one or other of the parents is absent. The attack usually starts with a sharp intake of breath as though the child were going to cry, but the cry never comes. The child's face may go red, then blue, and she may clench her teeth. The attack can be virtually aborted if you turn the child partially face down then gently place a finger over the back of the child's tongue and hook it forward so that she must involuntarily take a breath. Once you know you can deal with attacks you will stay calm and ten to one the attacks will become less frequent.

In the beginning it's easier said than done. Before I had children I used to find myself swearing that I would never tolerate the tantrums that I witnessed in my friends' children. Later I found myself making superhuman efforts to stay calm like every other parent who finds herself in public (worst of all with other competitive, unsympathetic parents who know it all) with a child in a tantrum. Rather than shame my son or myself I at first carried him from the room to a place where I could be alone with him and behave normally — instead of how I thought my friends expected me to behave — until we'd both regained our composure. Now with the confidence born of having been through it several times before, I lay them on the ground or floor a few feet from me and let them quieten down themselves. Just the other day my youngest son decided that his brothers' school field day was the place to pit his authority against mine. I laid him gently on the ground between serried ranks of proud parents and waited till the outburst was over. He was restored fairly quickly to his normal good humor because he had no one to fight with. I didn't get worked up, but transferred my attention to the sack race. An apparently snooty lady in front of me who had been viewing the antics of my youngest with disdain softened immediately and said it was the same with all her children. Her sympathy reassured and strengthened me — if only all parents could be as tolerant of one another!

13 The Working Mother

Mothers work for all sorts of reasons: from necessity, to contribute to the family income; from the desire to be independent and self-reliant; from boredom with the family and home; from the absolute personal *need* to work. As women have become freer to shape their own lives more and more mothers are working, and more and more simply because they enjoy it. They feel it enriches their lives, and if it does that it will certainly enrich family life. Until the last few years many women felt that it was their duty to ignore their own desires and serve the family. Now they feel acutely that they have the right to take their own wishes into consideration, and to make the decision to work even knowing that it will create difficulties for the family.

Many mothers possess the basic biological drive that makes them want to stay with and look after their children. Anything that takes them away from their children can be painful. The fundamental belief that it's wrong to desert the home and hearth for a job still haunts many women. Any question of doing so can raise doubts about whether they are good mothers, and feelings of guilt because their children must necessarily suffer some deprivation. Women with strong maternal instincts will be concerned not only with depriving their babies of affection, but also with their own sacrifices. These women crave the presence and company of their children (not *all* of the time, but much of the time) and especially when children are young it can be distressing to leave them even for a few hours. I well remember returning home from an important meeting that had gone on longer than I'd expected, when my second son was only a few days old. I had missed the four o'clock feeding and I drove madly along the highway, tears streaming down my face, to get back to my baby. My husband was taken aback at the passion that could elicit such frenzy. "I'm like a dog whining for her puppy," was as near as I could get to expressing how I felt in words.

There again you may be faced with a husband who has strong feelings about your returning to work, and his opinion must be considered too. In fact, it can only lead to unhappiness and resentment if you return to work and your partner is reluctant to see you do so. Your attitude may create friction between you and him, which will certainly affect the children. Discuss the matter, and see if you can reach a suitable compromise. The *quality* of life for the children when you are home is more important than the quantity, and constitutes an argument in favor of your going to work if the frustration you feel at being confined to domesticity makes you, your husband and the family unhappy. There are thousands of embittered women who feel the best years of their working lives were wasted on changing diapers and preparing meals. On the other hand, there are just as many who feel it is a privilege to give up the most satisfying job to tend their babies. You must do what is right for you and your family, in your own particular circumstances, and not be influenced by other people's opinions.

The Effect on Your Child

A good deal of research has been done in the last ten or fifteen years that no longer leaves open the questions of how a mother's absence affects her children and how important it is that the domestic atmosphere is happy and cheerful. The resolutions of both these questions are linked. If a mother stays at home to look after her children and thus becomes moody, resentful, and depressed, she may be actually doing her children a disservice by staying. For it has been shown that an unhappy mother at home can have a detrimental effect on her children, not to mention her husband, and can endanger a healthy family structure. Psychologists showed that children thrive best with two happy parents but do only marginally less well with *one* happy parent (of either sex). They don't do nearly as well with two unhappy parents and are in serious trouble with only one unhappy parent. So long as you and your husband are happy your children will do equally well whether you stay at home or go out to work.

A recent study that followed the progress of children of working mothers for seven years and compared their progress to a comparable group of children whose mothers did not work could only demonstrate one small difference between the two groups — the chil-

160

dren of working mothers had, on average, a slightly lower reading age than the other group. Physically, intellectually, emotionally and psychologically, as far as the tests could detect, the two groups of children were identical. There was an important proviso; the person acting as a substitute mother had to be attentive, loving and sympathetic. The sitter looking after a large number of children who was neglectful and impersonal, or who just didn't have the time to give each child individual attention, could not make up for a loving mother's absence and could adversely affect the development of the children in her care.

When to Start

Having decided that you are going to work after your baby is born, you must next establish when you will start, and you would be well advised to include your doctor in this decision. For there may be factors affecting your own health, and that of your baby, which should be considered and on which he can advise you. If you are going to breast-feed your baby this does not debar you from working, but you will have to find a job that allows you to take your baby with you and that provides some facilities for you to breast-feed. Some large companies have special nurseries where mothers can leave their babies of all ages with a trained nurse.

Much depends on how determined you are, because many obstacles can be overcome if you persevere. A doctor friend of mine was prepared to go to any lengths to work, have her baby with her and breast-feed him as well. Her job involved a good deal of travel but this did not deter her. He traveled with her everywhere. When he was very small he slept in a portable crib at her feet, and as he got older in a baby carriage in her office. She stopped whatever she was doing if he needed a feeding, and occasionally when she could not be with him she used a breast pump to withdraw her milk so that he never went without breast milk. Both thrived. *She* was perfectly happy, though often very tired, and *he* was just as happy being near his mother most of the time.

Not all of us have the energy, the perseverance or the guts to take on such a program. Even if you have not, one thing you must be prepared for if you are going to split your time and your loyalty between your family and your work is to be tired most evenings, sometimes utterly exhausted and now and then frustrated and anxious because neither your family nor your work is receiving your full attention. There's no doubt that it's hard — from all points of view. Having a husband who disagrees with what you're doing makes the strain unbearable, so do make an effort to come to terms with each other and understand each other's point of view. If the prospect of going back to work shortly after giving birth is deterring you from breast-feeding, take heart. All doctors agree that as little as two weeks of breast-feeding are very much better than no breast-feeding at all and give a baby a flying start. Try to organize your life so that you can do at least that.

You must also be fair to yourself. It is estimated that it takes about nine months for your metabolism to return to normal after a pregnancy. Parts of your body recover more quickly than others; if you menstruate three months after giving birth this is a good sign that your ovaries are getting back to their cyclical routine, but not all your hormone glands will be in step with them. The muscles, ligaments and joints that become more flexible and elastic to accommodate your pregnant shape and weight need to regain their tone and strength. Other vital organs like the heart, kidneys and lungs, together with your blood, gradually adjust to coping only with you and not with you plus the baby. If you have a responsible job it's important to wait until you are emotionally fit, so that your decision making is efficient. With all the changes going on in the body after pregnancy it's not surprising that women quickly feel tired, suffer aches and pains and get upset easily. Going back to work too early can only aggravate matters, so don't be precipitous. There's no hard and fast rule as to when you should take on a job — it depends on the individual person, her fortitude and her drives, but as a general rule few people should try to work before six weeks after delivery and then only part-time for about another six weeks. With my children I've been back in the office (though not full time) within a week of their birth and I would never repeat it. It's physically and emotionally too distressing. I would certainly never advise anyone to do it, but conversely I would never stop any mother from doing it because I sympathize with her impulse.

Benefits and Drawbacks

One of the aspects of being a working mother that makes life very hard is the necessity to invest all your free time in your family. In reality you're working at two jobs. Sometimes this is not too difficult. If, for instance, you have an intellectually taxing job you may have physical energy to spare when you get home for bath times, play, story reading and sympathetic listening. If, however, you're a teacher or a nurse, much of the sort of attention your children require will have been expended during your working day. Then it's doubly hard, but there's no escape. I firmly believe that a child, especially of preschool age, has the right to expect and receive his mother's attention when she is home from work. The price of this is high. Instead of dropping your coat and pouring yourself a drink you'll have to pick up the baby and do everything else one-handed until he's asleep. Instead of climbing into a bath to soothe your shattered nerves, you'll have to cope with the children's bath time and games. Instead of settling down with the newspaper you'll have to read bedtime stories. After they are settled and asleep you can start thinking about an evening meal. When you do finally fall asleep, ten to one your night will be disturbed. You don't have to be generous of spirit, you have to be sacrificial and so does your husband. Don't forget him — you will both need attention and understanding.

While you are bound to think sometimes that your children are getting a raw deal, it's reassuring that when children are young they accept their lives as the norm. Will, my third son, returned from his first day at nursery school babbling about his new friend Gavin, whose Mummy was a doctor. "Is she really a doctor?" I asked. "Well, Mummies *are* doctors," was his reply. My four sons don't turn a hair when their mother has to dash off to foreign parts for a few days to attend a conference — don't all Mums do that? The length of time spent without their mother counts far less with children than the *quality* of the time spent with her. Love isn't measured in time. Love is what you put into time, no matter how short.

Who's Going to Look After Your Child?

It's not surprising that women make good administrators. Running a home requires a good organizer; running a home and a job requires something of an organizing genius. But even an organizing genius needs help. If your job is a full-time one you will certainly need someone to help take care of the children. An experienced nanny is ideal, but of course few of us can afford that. Mothers, mothers-in-law and relatives are marvelous for helping out in the short term, but you will feel you cannot make the demands on them that you can on someone you employ. Even before I was married and had children, I used to promise myself that even if my salary only covered the cost of having a nanny, I would nevertheless go out to work. I still believe this. And if there is enough in the kitty, everyone in the family will benefit from certain other chores being taken off your shoulders. A housekeeper two or three times a week is an investment you will never regret.

If you opt for a sitter, try to get one who will come to your own house — your baby will be happier on home ground than in a strange house. If the person runs a nursery, make sure you visit it and see the rooms and facilities. Have a long chat with your prospective mother-substitute and try to establish what sort of person she is and what her methods are. Many sitters are excellent, but some do the minimum for your child. In this atmosphere the child cannot flourish. If you have any doubts, look further.

Not everyone can afford this kind of help, but whatever sort of help you have, be it a nanny or a neighbor, it's up to individual members of the family to help out. If both parents are working, I think it's essential that the father does his share and this must be understood. Sharing cooking, doing the dishes, cleaning, laundering, diaper changing and the countless other household tasks are surely part of a modern marriage. Older children must help out too. In institutions children are well able to set the table at four, make their own beds at five, serve a simple cold breakfast at six, be trusted to watch over youngsters for a while at seven, run errands at eight and help with anything at nine if supervised. Why not at home? If necessary, jobs should be allocated. Qualities of helpfulness, patience, consideration and thoughtfulness should not just be encouraged but accepted as the normal way of life from an early age. Most children have an acute desire to help from the time that they can walk and bring small things for you. They wish to be given responsibility. If their efforts are praised and rewarded, even the most truculent children can become useful and pleasant members of the household. By the age of six, the majority of children understand the value of fair play, and they often respond if you explain that something done for them deserves reciprocation. Participation in the day-to-day activities of the home encourages self-assurance, self-reliance and, like all of us, children get a kick out of being part of a team, especially when it works well.

14 Contraception

When to Start Again

There's a generally held belief that it's impossible to conceive while you're breast-feeding your baby. It is true that the hormone that stimulates secretion of milk has an inhibitory effect on ovulation, but it is by no means 100 percent safe. Many women relying on lactation as a foolproof method of contraception have found themselves pregnant four or five months after giving birth to a baby. There is no fixed time for the ovaries to get back to their normal cyclic activity, but about half of all mothers have ovulated (and menstruated) by the fourth month after delivery. So you must start thinking about contraception before you have your six-week checkup. It takes a surprisingly long time for your body to get back to normal after a pregnancy (about nine months), so you will in any case not really be fit enough, strong enough or emotionally stable enough to contemplate pregnancy before this. I also think that your baby should enjoy at least a year of being the baby in the family, even if you want another child fairly quickly. At your six-week visit you can discuss with your doctor the various contraceptive methods that are available. You may want a change from the contraceptive method you used before having your baby, or you may perhaps not know too much about the subject anyway. Either way, now is the time to get it all organized.

There are a variety of methods open to you which can be suited to your taste and need. Some methods, like the oral contraceptive pill, are virtually infallible if taken as instructed but carry with them side effects of which you must be aware. Others, like the sheath or diaphragm, have few hazards linked to their use but their effectiveness is considerably less than the pill. So if you are anxious not to conceive it's important that you choose the most effective method and you will probably decide that the small risk associated with that method is worth taking. If all you want to do is space your family you may be happy to accept a method with a higher failure rate. There may be medical reasons that have an important bearing on your choice; for instance, if you've already had a deep vein thrombosis of the leg you should not take an oral contraceptive containing estrogen because of the small associated risk of a further thrombosis.

Today we are fortunate in having a wide range of contraceptives. Here are some of them.

Natural: Rhythm method
Mechanical: Sheath, Diaphragm, Intrauterine device (IUD)
Chemical: Spermicidal jellies and cream
Hormonal: Estrogen/progestogen oral contraceptive, Progestogen-only oral contraceptive
Mechanical/Hormonal: Progestogen-containing IUD
Surgical: Vasectomy, Tubal tie, Hysterectomy, Termination

Natural Method

This method relies on abstaining from intercourse during the time around ovulation. In most women ovulation occurs about the fourteenth day (counting the first day of bleeding as the first day of the cycle). To allow for a late or early ovulation you should avoid intercourse from the twelfth to the seventeenth day. It's quite an easy job to find out exactly when you are ovulating by taking your temperature each day. Many observant women have learned other telltale signs such as ovulation headache or slight discomfort on the right or left side of the abdomen. If you record your temperature every morning for a month you will see that on the fourteenth day, approximately, it rises a little and remains raised for the rest of the month. Keeping a chart like the one opposite will confirm your own pattern of ovulation. Once you have established your regular pattern you can abstain from intercourse appropriately.

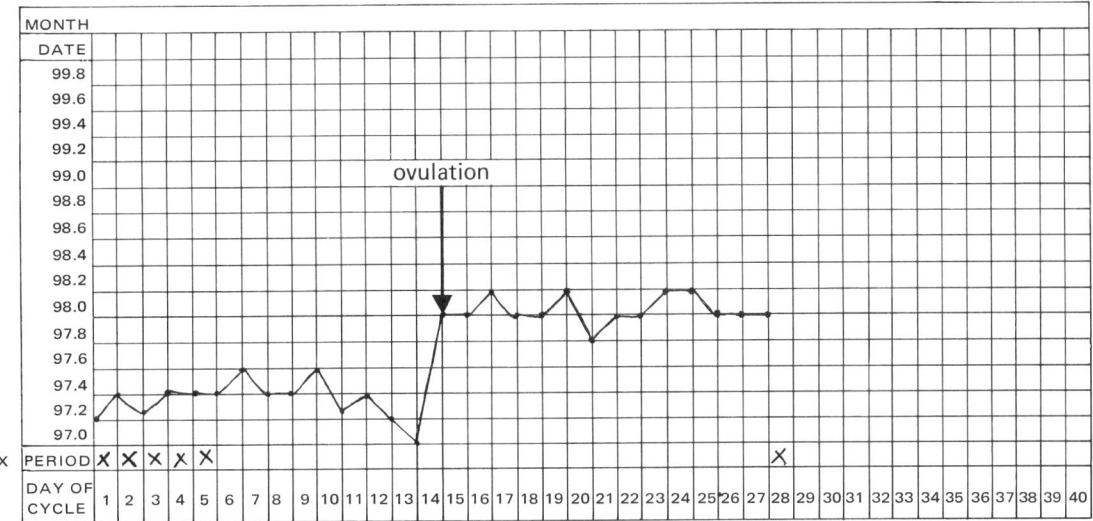

X Put a cross for each day of period.

Mark the temperature by a dot in the appropriate square.

Mechanical Methods

SHEATH

The sheath and the diaphragm work by mechanically preventing the sperm from reaching the ovum, and so prohibit fertilization. With the sheath worn over the man's penis, the sperm never even enter the woman's body. Many couples, however, find this method aesthetically unacceptable.

DIAPHRAGM

If a vaginal diaphragm is used, the sperm enter the vagina but are trapped there, and cannot penetrate the cervical canal or reach the ovum. It is advisable to use a spermicidal cream or jelly in conjunction with a diaphragm. You run a small amount all round the rim, not forgetting a good measure in the middle of the cap, on the surface that touches the cervix. In careful hands, this method is fairly successful and can be quite aesthetically acceptable to some women if you think of it as a nightly habit, like brushing your teeth. A variation of the vaginal diaphragm is the cervical cap, which fits snugly over the cervix and requires a bit of practice before you can fit it efficiently.

INTRAUTERINE DEVICE (IUD)

The intrauterine device works in quite a different way from the sheath and the diaphragm, as it actually allows fertilization to take place. For over one hundred years we've known that a 'foreign body' lodged inside the cavity of the uterus would discourage pregnancy. IUDs were first used in 1800 and in the past all sorts of materials were tried. Now, for the most part, we use small flexible plastic devices that are introduced into the uterus under sterile conditions. Plastic is inert and doesn't therefore have any direct effect on the functioning of the uterus. IUDs work by making the womb 'irritable' (it contracts very readily) so that a fertilized ovum isn't allowed to implant. The menstrual cycle proceeds normally, the fertilized ovum dies and is expelled at the end of the month in the menstrual flow. Many women find IUDs quite acceptable. Others experience pain during or after insertion, or on intercourse. Others find that bleeding at period time becomes much heavier; still others expel the device; vaginal discharge is quite common and very rarely an ectopic pregnancy (the baby develops in a Fallopian tube and this pregnancy must be terminated by a surgical operation) occurs. Most IUDs are unsuitable for women who have not borne children and should not be fitted to women who already have very heavy periods or an infection of the uterus. If you find an IUD suitable you should see your doctor once a year for a checkup. It's a measure of the success of IUDs that 50 percent of women fitted with them are still using them at the end of six years.

Chemical Methods

There are a variety of jellies, pastes, creams and pessaries available which are lethal to sperm and if used in the vagina provide a chemical barrier against sperm reaching the ovum. Spermicides may be used alone, though it is unwise to rely on them completely as the failure rate is quite high. They may be used as supplements to other methods, for instance with the diaphragm or sheath. The amount normally necessary is 0.07 ounces (2 grams) or a three- to four-inch (7.5–10 centimeter) ribbon of cream. If intercourse is repeated more of the spermicide should be used.

The latest type of spermicide is the 'C-film.' It is a square of water-soluble plastic which has been impregnated with a potent spermicide and in laboratory trials has been found satisfactory. It is truly unisex and can be used by either partner. Even with the most careful use it does not approach the effectiveness of the oral contraceptive.

Hormonal Methods

Many women and their partners find oral contraceptives the most aesthetically acceptable method of birth control because taking the pill is unrelated to intercourse. It's therefore doubly important to take the pill regularly and it's best to put your pack of pills in a place where you will see it every day. Your pill can be taken at any time of day but forgetting to take it for twenty-four hours can lower its efficiency, particularly with the low-dose estrogen pill. There are two main types of hormonal contraceptive pill: those that contain both female hormones (estrogen and progestogen in synthetic forms that closely mimic the natural hormone) — the 'combined' pill — and those that contain only progestogen. They work in different ways and have slightly different failure rates.

The combined pills work by suppressing ovulation. As an egg is not dropped and therefore is not available for fertilization each month, this method has the lowest failure rate. The course of tablets is usually started on the fifth day of bleeding and is taken each day for twenty-one days. A period usually follows three or four days after taking the last pill of the pack.

As the name implies, the progestogen-only pill contains no estrogen and is virtually free of the side effects associated with taking estrogens. It is a useful method for a woman who wants to take an oral contraceptive for convenience but who feels reluctant to take estrogens or who, in her doctor's opinion, has good medical reasons not to.

The progestogen-only pill works in quite a different way from the combined pill, but there are more pregnancies in women taking

169

it. It probably acts by making the mucus in the cervical canal so thick and hostile that sperm cannot penetrate it to reach the body of the uterus. It also has some action on the lining of the womb, making it unreceptive to the ovum if it does by chance get fertilized. Thirdly, it probably has a direct effect on the sperm itself, making it less capable of fertilizing an ovum.

This pill is not free of side effects. The main drawbacks are irregular bleeding, which normally settles down after the first few months, and subsequent, though rarely permanent, amenorrhea (loss of periods). Nevertheless the progestogen-only pill is a good alternative for women who cannot take the combined oral contraceptive. And it can be very effective if the instructions are followed carefully.

The oral contraceptive pill is still a subject of confusion and sensationalism about the risks associated with it, and many women who are trying to decide if they should start using the pill have questions to ask. Quite rightly they want to have the facts. Most of the oral contraceptive manufacturers print explanatory patient booklets that will answer many of your questions and put side-effects into perspective. Whatever method of contraception you and your partner are considering, discuss the whole subject with your doctor, who will advise you according to your individual needs. If you opt for the contraceptive pill, make sure you understand the implications of its use. And remember, no one should take the pill without her doctor's knowledge. There are many oral contraceptive pills available in the United States containing different synthetic hormones in different amounts, so there should be one that suits you. Make sure you go and see your doctor for a routine checkup three months after starting an oral contraceptive, again at six months, and then every six months after that.

Mechanical/Hormonal Method

One of the newest contraceptive devices is an IUD that contains progestogen. Theoretically this device should be very effective, as it will combine the efficacy of the IUD and the progestogen-only pill. In addition it is claimed that it delivers the progestogen only to the place where it is needed — that is, the uterus and cervix — and should therefore have few side effects. This device should compare favorably both in safety and efficacy with other types of contraceptives.

Surgical Methods

There is no more reliable method of preventing pregnancy than male and female sterilization. As we have no sure way of reversing this operation, it must be considered permanent.

VASECTOMY

Vasectomy involves dividing and usually removing a portion of the vas deferens so that discontinuity is assured. The vas deferens is a muscular tube that transports sperm from the testes to the seminal vesicles situated underneath the bladder where they are stored. It is essential that both partners are happy about the operation before it is carried out. Prior to consenting, husband and wife should discuss all the implications of vasectomy with their doctor or surgeon. As there is little chance of restoring the patency of the duct, the operation should be considered irreversible. For this reason vasectomy appeals most to middle-aged couples whose family is complete and whose marriage is stable. After the operation, it is necessary to examine specimens of semen at monthly intervals. Not until two sperm-free specimens have been obtained may the man regard himself as infertile.

Intercourse can usually be resumed a few days after the operation and it is important that ejaculation is reestablished. As viable sperm can be released from the seminal vesicles for several months, alternative methods of contraception must be used until the semen is sperm free. The operation does not affect the testes and the enjoyment of intercourse and normal ejaculation should continue with no loss of potency.

Vasectomy can be performed under local or general anesthetic. It is a simple, quick job for the surgeon and either way the patient has no need to stay in the hospital.

STERILIZATION OF THE WOMAN

The operation to sterilize a woman may necessitate a general anesthetic and a week to ten days in the hospital. A woman is sterilized by cutting and tying the Fallopian tubes, which, with modern techniques, may not even involve opening the abdominal cavity. Many female sterilizations are done when a Caesarean section is performed. As with vasectomy the patient, her husband and her general practitioner must all consent to the operation.

HYSTERECTOMY

Hysterectomy is rarely performed for contraceptive purposes alone. It is usually considered only if there are sound medical reasons. Subtotal hysterectomy leaves the ovaries intact, while total hysterectomy involves the removal of the ovaries as well as the uterus. In the latter case treatment with hormone supplements is often needed postoperatively in a premenopausal woman.

TERMINATION

With the development of new techniques it is possible to perform termination without a general anesthetic. Despite recent advances, termination of pregnancy carries with it significant risks. More widespread and more efficient contraception would help reduce these hazards; prevention of conception will always be preferable to termination.

Comparative Efficiency of Various Methods

Comparing the failure rates of different contraceptive methods can help partners decide which contraceptive method will best suit them. The efficiency of any one method depends not only on its own reliability but also on its acceptability to an individual couple and the fertility of that couple.

The efficiency of a method is expressed in a universally accepted notation — the number of pregnancies per hundred 'woman years' of use. Most women ovulate monthly and therefore there are twelve opportunities in a year for conception. So the efficiency is

$$\frac{\text{The number of pregnancies} \times 12 \times 100}{\text{months of use}}$$

So if four pregnancies occur in eight-thousand cycles (or months) the efficiency will be

$$\frac{4 \times 12 \times 100}{8000} = 0.60 \text{ (this is a theoretical figure)}$$

This value or index for different methods can be compared and will give a good idea of relative efficiency. A very simple example of how the efficiency index is used will show you its significance. If the failure rate of a method is one, this means that of one hundred women using that method for a year one will become pregnant. Here are failure rates for various methods:

Method	Failure Rate
Oral contraceptives	less than 1 (0.34)
a. estrogen containing	2.0
b. estrogen free	2.4
Intrauterine device (IUD)	2.8–7.5
Condom	6.0
Rhythm (by temperature chart)	7.2
Diaphragm and spermicide	23.5
Spermicides alone	

Contraception, whatever form you decide on, should be used for what it is — a means to an end. It is a means by which couples can space their families according to their emotional, domestic, and financial considerations. Just as important, it is a means by which couples can contain their families to the number of children they really do want. And probably most important, contraception is a means by which a woman can take the initiative and decide both if and when she is going to become pregnant. We acknowledge this initiative as a fundamental freedom to be enjoyed by all women — basic mother care, which is the first essential of baby care.

Glossary

Amenorrhea Absence or abnormal stoppage of the menstrual period.

Amniocentesis The passage of an instrument to the cavity of the uterus through the abdominal wall to take a specimen of amniotic fluid.

Amniotic fluid The fluid that surrounds the developing embryo inside its sac.

Analgesic An agent that alleviates pain without causing loss of consciousness.

Androgen Any substance that possesses masculinizing activity, a male hormone.

Antipyretic An agent that relieves or reduces fever.

Cervix The neck of the uterus.

Chloasma A discoloration of the skin occurring in yellowish brown patches and pimples.

Coitus Sexual union between individuals of the opposite sex.

Colostrum The thin milky fluid formed by the breasts before or just after labor.

Conception The fertilization of the ovary.

Curettage The removal of material from the cavity of the uterus by scraping.

Douche A stream of water (gas or vapor) directed against part of the body or into a cavity.

Dysmenorrhea Painful menstruation.

Embryo The developing product of fertilization of an ovary.

Episiotomy Surgical incision of the vaginal opening for obstetric purposes.

Ergometrine A drug that stimulates the uterus to contract down and remain contracted.

Estrogen Hormone produced by the ovary in the first half of the menstrual cycle resulting in ovulation.

Fallopian tube The tube that extends from the upper part of either side of the uterus to the ovary.

Fertilization The fusion of a sperm with an ovum.

Fetus The developing embryo or baby.

Folic acid One of the B vitamins.

Gamma globulin A type of protein that can be used in the prevention of certain infectious diseases if given as a sterile solution containing antibodies normally present in adult human blood, i.e. as an immunizing agent.

Gynecology The branch of medicine that treats diseases of the genital tract in women.

Hemoglobin The oxygen carrying pigment of the red blood cells.

Hormone The chemical substance produced in one part of the body and transported in the bloodstream to another organ where the effect is produced.

Malocclusion An abnormality of the contact made by the upper and lower teeth.

Membrane A thin layer of tissue that usually covers the surface of an organ or divides a space.

Menstruate The passage of blood from the genital tract at monthly intervals.

Obstetrics The branch of surgery that deals with the management of pregnancy, labor and the puerperium.

Ovulation The discharge of a mature ovum from the surface of the ovary.

Ovum An egg.

Oxytocin A hormone that stimulates contraction of the uterus.

Pediatrician A physician who specializes in the treatment of diseases in children (up to and including 12 years of age).

Placenta The cake-like organ within the uterus which establishes communication between the mother and child by means of the umbilical cord.

Prenatal Occurring or formed before birth.

Progesterone The hormone produced by the ovary during the second part of the cycle which prepares the uterus for the reception and development of the fertilized ovum.

Postpartum Occurring after childbirth or after delivery.

Puerperium The period after labor.

Sperm A mature male cell produced in the testis which can impregnate the ovum.

Testis (pl. *testes*) The male genital organ that manufactures sperm and male hormones.

Uterus The hollow muscular organ in females that is the place of nourishment of the embryo and fetus.

Vernix A creamy, greasy substance that covers the skin of the fetus.

Index

182

oral contraceptives containing estrogen and (combined pill), 169, 173
oral contraceptives containing only (estrogen-free oral contraceptives), 169–170, 173
Punishment, 151
Pus, coming from ear, 115
Pyloric stenosis, 81

Quarantine, 122
Questions, answering children's, 136–138

Rashes
  diaper, 76–77, 84
  infected, 77
  infectious disease and, 120, 122
  in newborn babies, 76–77
  See also Eczema
Reading, 146–147
Reading age, 161
Reading materials, 147
Reciprocation, understanding of, 164
Relationships, *see* Friends; Parent-child relationship; Parents, relationship between; Personal relationships
Relatives, 133
  See also Grandparents
Reproductive system, female, 7
Requests
  crying as communication of, 65, 132–133
  See also Demands
Respiratory tract, upper: infections of, 113–115
Responsibility, giving children, 164
Rest
  during first few weeks after delivery, 47, 68, 69
  during pregnancy, 14–15

Reward, 134
Rhesus incompatibility, 77–78
Rhythm method (natural method of contraception; monitoring menstrual cycle), 4, 166–167, 173
Ringworm, 125
Rocking movements, 153
Room temperature, *see* Temperature (of surroundings)
Roughage, 109, 118
Routine
  baby as responsive to, 69
  feeding, 54–55
Rubella, *see* German measles
Rules, 150

Scalp, scales on (cradle cap), 74
School, introduction to nursery, 135–136
"Security blankets," 154
Sex (gender), determining baby's, 4–5
Sex (sexual intercourse)
  children's questions about, 136–137
  during pregnancy, 16
  after vasectomy, 171
Sex education, 137
Sex organs, 88, 91, 137
  See also Penis
Sheath (condom), 165, 167, 173
Sheets, 108, 152
Siblings (other children), baby's arrival and reaction of, 46–47
Sitter, working mother and, 161, 164
Sitting, 94–95
Skin
  of newborn baby, 45–46, 74–75
  during pregnancy, 24
  See also Jaundice

Tests
  for fetal abnormalities, 27
  for pregnancy, 14
  prenatal, 25, 78
Tetanus, immunization against,
  128
Thermometers, 123
Thrombosis, oral contraceptives
  and, 166
Thrush, 84
Thumb-sucking, 55, 154
Time
  children's sense of, 151
  free, for mother, 68–69
Tiredness
  crying and, 67
  of working mother, 161–162
Toilet training, *see* Bladder
  control; Bowel control
Tongue-tie, 83
Tonsillitis, acute, 115
Tonsils, 113–115
Tooth decay, 127
Toothbrush, 127
Towels, 28
  wrapping the baby in, 45
Training pants, 108
Transfusion, for rhesus
  incompatibility, 78
Transitoriness, law of, 141
Travel, during pregnancy, 15
Truthfulness, 136, 138, 155
Tuberculosis, immunization
  against, 129
Twins, 26–27, 52

Ulcers, mouth, 118–119
Umbilical cord, separation of, 46,
  82
Understanding
  learning and, 90–91
  reasons for parental requests,
  150

Upper respiratory tract infection,
  113–115
Urination, *see* Bladder control
Urticaria, 76, 126–127

Vaccination, *see* Immunization
Vagina, cutting of (episiotomy), 35
Varicose veins, during pregnancy,
  25
Vasectomy, 171
Veins
  thrombosis, 166
  varicose, 25
Verbalization
  importance of, 136
  See also Speaking
Verrucae, 125
Vitamin and mineral supplements,
  during pregnancy, 17–18
Vitamin C, 59, 60
Vitamin drops, 59–60, 62
Vomiting, 111, 117
  of newborn babies, 80–81
  during pregnancy, 19, 22

Waking the baby, for feeding, 54–
  55, 59
Walking, 98–99
Warts, 125
Washing
  fontanelle, 74
  See also Bathing; Cleansing;
  Sponging
Water, boiled, 44, 58, 59, 67, 82
Water games, 145
Watering eyes, 79
Waters, breaking of the, 33
Weight, 85–86
Weight gain
  in babies, 63 (*see also* Fat
  accumulation)
  during pregnancy, 22–23, 27
Weight loss, breast-feeding and,
  50–51

Dr. Miriam Stoppard

has written extensively on child-related topics for British journals and magazines, and contributes a weekly column on baby care to the London *Evening News*. She practiced as a doctor for eight years before joining a major pharmaceutical company, of which she is now deputy managing director. She lives with her husband, playwright Tom Stoppard, and family in Buckinghamshire, England.